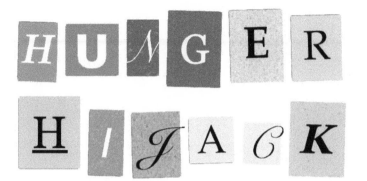

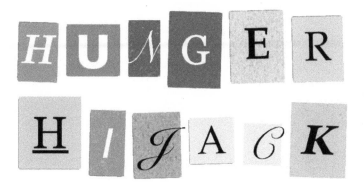

# HUNGER HIJACK

How your eating habits are changing
your brain and making you sick

## David Sherer MD

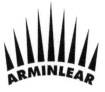

ARMINLEAR

Library of Congress Control Number: 2024931868

ISBN (paperback): 978-1-963271-09-6
(eBook): 978-1-963271-10-2

Armin Lear Press, Inc.
215 W Riverside Drive, #4362
Estes Park, CO 80517

*This book is dedicated to LBS*

# CONTENTS

# DISCLAIMER

This book is for information purposes only and is not intended to diagnose, treat, or cure any disease, affliction, or medical condition. Always consult with your personal doctor and health care team before changing any medical regimen.

"Let food be thy medicine ..."

**Attributed to Hippocrates**

# AUTHOR'S NOTE

On the night of December 8, 1982, when I was a third-year medical student in Boston, I received a call from my brother who had told me that our 27-year-old sister Lisa had died that day from complications related to juvenile diabetes. First diagnosed at age 7, Lisa had endured a long and rough path with her disease. Known to be a "brittle diabetic," that is, one whose blood sugar was difficult to control, Lisa nonetheless graduated from college and was in graduate school studying social work when she became gravely ill. By the time she was in her early twenties, she was experiencing many of the complications of her pathology, including almost complete blindness, kidney failure, nerve damage and incontinence, and a failed kidney transplant. When most people her age were in the prime of their lives, she was riddled with disease. Three days prior to her death she had told me by telephone that she had "had enough" and was going to stop her insulin therapy. I didn't believe her.

On the morning of August 27, 2007, almost a quarter century after my sister had died, I spoke to my diabetic father on the telephone from his hospital room where he was being treated for pneumonia. It would turn out to be the last conversation I had with him, for shortly thereafter I received a call from the doctor caring for him that he had passed away later that morning. His course with diabetes was quite different from his daughter's in that he lived to what we call a "ripe old age" (87) and apparently suffered few if any of the devastating complications of diabetes that my sister had. He had remained fairly active near the end of his life – traveling, playing golf, and living life on his own terms.

For the past 25 years I have been on a crusade to warn people about the dangers, despite current popular sentiment, inherent to overweight/obesity and the consumption of diets rich in saturated fat, sugar, and refined carbohydrates and ultra-processed foods (UPF). I am not the first to discuss these issues, nor will I be the last. I mention this because the incidence and prevalence of diabetes has skyrocketed across the world. Increasing body mass index and UPF have both been implicated as major contributors to what we are seeing as emerging trends of human disease, particularly type 2 diabetes, cardiovascular disease, and cancer.

Admittedly, juvenile diabetes (type 1) is a very different disease than adult onset, or type 2 diabetes, but the potential endpoint is much the same: a relative or absolute deficiency of insulin, sometimes associated with a resistance to the action of existing systemic insulin. Acutely, absence of insulin without supplementation is fatal, and its lack can eventually lead to organ and tissue damage.

My hope is that through knowledge, people can see the dangers and help themselves before it is too late.

For convenience sake, I will sometimes refer to processed foods rich in saturated fat, refined carbohydrates, sugar, and salt as *bad food*. This bad food appellation also applies to most ultra-processed food (UPF). Not all UPF is rich in saturated fat, refined carbohydrates, sugar, and salt, just as not all food rich in saturated fat, refined carbohydrates, sugar, and salt is UPF. Physician Chris Van Tulleken, whom I reference frequently in this book, has quoted a recognized definition of UPF as "Formulations of ingredients, mostly of exclusive industrial use, made by a series of industrial processes, many requiring sophisticated equipment and technology." To me, UPF is almost always bad food, as is food high in saturated fat, refined carbohydrates, white sugar, and salt. The term bad food is imperfect, but it gets the point across.

# INTRODUCTION

"If you put junk food into your body,
your body will turn to junk."

**Goldie Hawn, actress**

In the early part of the spring of 2020, when the Covid-19 pandemic was just gaining steam, I was conducting some research for another book I was writing and came across a past article from *Forbes* magazine that piqued my interest. The article, entitled "The New Theory On Weight Loss: Your Bad Diet Has Damaged Your Brain" was written by *Forbes* contributor Melanie Haiken, and it first appeared on August 21, 2013. In the article the author presented startling evidence found by scientists at the University of Liverpool in the UK. She revealed:

> "What they found was that a diet high in saturated fat
> and simple carbohydrates sets in motion a chain reaction
> of 'metabolic dysfunction' involving the appetite regu-
> lating hormones leptin and ghrelin. (Leptin's job is to

suppress appetite, ghrelin's to increase it.) In addition, a fatty high-carb diet resulted in 'alterations in structural plasticity' – i.e. brain changes."

As a physician for over four decades, this revelation intrigued me. The idea that the majority of foods we eat today – foods mostly associated with what has been referred to as the "Western diet" (though this diet is not now merely confined to the West but has spread it's tentacles all over the world) – are causing physical changes in our brains. These changes, occurring primarily in the appetite center of the brain, the hypothalamus, are altering our perception of hunger and satiety (fullness) and leading us down the path, unwittingly and insidiously, toward overweight, obesity and all the dangerous health conditions that go along with that.

Haiken had interviewed an expert in the field of weight and obesity for the article, Dr. Louis Aronne of the Comprehensive Weight-Control Program at New York-Presbyterian Hospital/ Weill Cornell Medical Center. He spoke with her about the conundrum that faces so many people today. She asked, "Why do some people seem to find it impossible to lose weight, despite numerous serious attempts to get slim using diet and exercise?"

Aronne gave her a simple answer, with specific reference to the foods we eat:

> "The evidence is quite convincing – eating fattening foods causes inflammatory cells to go into the hypo- thalamus . . . This overloads the neurons and causes neurological damage."

Analyzing the data and relying on what Aronne had told her, Haiken summarized her discoveries and Aronne's core message:

"In other words, your brain has gone haywire and you can no longer trust the messages it's sending you about appetite, hunger and fullness. 'It's like your gas gauge points to empty all the time, whether or not the tank is full.' says Aronne."

Aronne, whose work is so important in these times, is evidently fond of saying "It's about biology . . . If less fatty food comes in, it reduces the rate of damage (to the hypothalamus)." Haiken adds that, according to Aronne's sentiments, ". . . it doesn't matter so much which specific diet you follow, as long as it's one that cuts calories, reduces fat, and reduces simple carbohydrates."

After I had read this article, so many things began to make sense regarding the overweight/obesity epidemic that is rampant in the United States and is sweeping the world. In the U.S., an astounding 70 percent of people are either overweight (having a body mass index of greater than 25) or obese (having a body mass index of greater than 30). Hand in glove with this is the dramatic rise in diabetes. The Center for Disease Control reports that 38.4 million people, 11.6 percent of the population, have diabetes and 8.7 million people have it and don't even know it. As worrisome still is the number of people with pre-diabetes, a condition that may lead to actual diabetes itself, where 97.6 million aged 18 years or older suffer from it. Additionally, 27.2 million adults over 65 have pre-diabetes. The CDC goes on to say that in 2022, it cost the U.S. 413 billion USD in direct and indirect medical costs to treat diabetes. And as I explore later, diabetes is merely the tip of the iceberg when it comes to diseases associated with being overweight or obese.

When you do the math, it is not hard to see that in a nation of about 330 million people, well over one-third of Americans are either diabetic or pre-diabetic. This is a very dangerous situation, both from a health perspective and a financial one. For if these numbers stay at the same level or continue their rise (as they likely will), the financial burden on the United States may become untenable. In 2021, US healthcare expenditure reached 4.3 trillion USD, or about 12,914 USD per person. This represented about 18.3 percent of the US Gross Domestic Product and a growth of 2.7 percent from the prior year. Combined with the critical shortages of primary care physicians, nurses, and other health care workers, and the fact that more people are turning 65 by the year 2030 than at any point in our nation's history, a perfect storm is brewing that will severely challenge the healthcare delivery model for the U.S. This storm, a mere six years off on the horizon, will test the nation morally, financially and – for you – personally. It is a frightening prospect to contemplate. As I often say in my writings and lectures, we have not merely a healthcare crisis in our midst but a *health crisis*.

The information in the *Forbes* article that so intrigued me was only part of the story, as I soon discovered. For in reality, the research shows that overweight and obesity in and of themselves do not fully account for the health risks we face today with regard to what and how we eat. As it turns out, a parallel phenomenon is occurring that has as much and perhaps even more significance to this story, and that is ultra processed food, or UPF.

But before I go any further, I must state something vitally important. *My book is not intended to judge, shame, or otherwise label anyone who struggles with weight. Each person is an individual of infinite worth, with a unique backstory and set of life circumstances.* Rather, the intent of this work is to enlighten you about the science behind why body mass index has risen so dramatically in many parts of the globe in the last five decades, and what that means for our health, many nations' economies, and indeed the Earth's environment. Interestingly, it also has implications for the military readiness and defense of many countries, especially that of the United States.

This book, in which I have somewhat of a personal stake, has been on my mind for many years and the article in *Forbes* was just the catalyst I needed to spark a focused investigation. As a physician and the son of a groundbreaking NIH trained endocrinologist, whose sibling of a sister who lost her life at age 27 to juvenile diabetes, I had often wondered how it came to be that so many people in my own country and, indeed the world, have become so overweight. I came to realize that at the very core of this problem lays an approach to overweight/obesity and its health ramifications that is not adequately considered when discussing this issue, and that is the issue of addiction.

Addiction, just like the prevalence of obesity and the presence of UPF, is widespread in the world and growing. Whether to caffeine, electronic devices, pornography, illicit drugs, alcohol, cigarettes, or any other entity you might choose, it is my contention that addiction figures prominently when examining the world's weight challenges and concomitant health problems. Because of my desire to present relevant material in a simple and easy way to remember I have structured this book in a format as simple as **A, B, C**, and **D**.

**A** stands for **A**ddiction, the underpinning, I believe, of science elucidated at the University of Liverpool (and many other places, as we shall see) and what Dr. Aronne so convincingly articulates in his work.

**B** represents **B**ackground and **B**enefit, meaning both the backstory of how we came to this point as a human society (and a personal accounting of my own habits), and which commercial entities have benefited from the changes in our collective brains to the tune of trillions of dollars.

**C** means **C**omplications and **C**onsequences, the things that have resulted, health-wise, fiscally, climate-wise, and in other ways more subtle, from the problem as well as the diseases that directly or indirectly emerge from overweight/obesity.

**D**, stands for what do we **D**o about it, both personally and as a society.

When I speak and write about the sensitive topic of body weight, I am often accused of being insensitive or, in contemporary parlance, fat-shaming. My answer to that is simple: Science beats sentiment every time. The reason I have such strong conviction in this is that I've seen, in 40+ years in medicine, the ravages to health a high body mass index can bring. Is it shaming to tell a cigarette smoker to quit, or a user of illicit drugs to get addiction help? For me, approaching the problem under discussion here is no different. The fact that fifty years ago the average adult male in the United States weighed 150 pounds as compared to 200 pounds today is all too telling. Clearly our habits and our adulterated food has driven our altered brains – not genetics, poor metabolism, or any other alleged mitigating factor one might choose – toward impaired health. Said another way, our problem is *what we eat*, not *who we are* as individuals.

Much of my research has come from three sources: scholarly articles that are evidenced based, (that is, backed by the scientific method and peer reviewed), articles from the mainstream press, and insightful writings from authors such as former Food and Drug Administration director David Kessler, journalist Michael Moss, and physician Chris Van Tulleken. I ask your indulgence as you read because you will find many references to support my views. I have tried to choose the most compelling research articles to get my point across; there is so much evidence out there that it is a challenge in curating just the right literature to prove a point. Do realize though that some of the evidence does not in every case prove *causality* but instead points to *correlation and association*. But sometimes in scientific inquiry these types of evidence are all we have in the search for truth. But as the saying goes, "Where there's smoke, there's fire."

For the health of our nation and indeed the world the time has come to speak plainly, sensitively, and respectfully. Our futures might literally depend upon it. When you read what I have to say bear in mind that certain recurring themes run through the narrative. When you look carefully at the combined science related to human biologic illness, body weight, processed food, and physical inactivity, you notice that consistent reference is made to inflammation, oxidative stress, autoimmunity and damage to the bacteria composition and function in our digestive systems. I do my best to explain these concepts, which in their aggregate (as they relate to human disease) strike me as being akin to Albert Einstein's quest for a unified field theory of fundamental forces in the physical world.

The watchword for what I believe underlies the explosion of

human disease in our times is "artificial." The Merriam Webster definition of artificial is "lacking in natural quality," "imitation, sham" or "based on differential morphological characters not necessarily indicative of natural relationships." Today we have so much that has been deemed "artificial": our food has artificial ingredients and flavorings, the buzzword in the tech world is artificial intelligence (AI), our soft drinks have artificial sweeteners, our movies use computer-generated imagery to create artificial images, and politicians of a certain stripe claim that whatever goes against their image, narrative, and opinion is "fake news" (that is, artificial news).

Because so much of what we are exposed to in our physical lives is artificial, I think we have a tension – a *clash* if you will – that exists between our human biology and synthetically created elements present in the modern world. That clash is, in my opinion, representative of the battle being fought on both a micro and macro level. On the micro level we see disease forming because of direct and indirect physiologic effects of molecules that did not exist even one hundred years ago. It is as if our bodies and immune systems don't know what to make of these substances. On the macro level we are suffering the gradual warming of the planet and, for the first time in history, the real prospect of complete planetary destruction due to pollution, climate change and the prospect of nuclear, biological, and chemical warfare. We also see a macro result not many in the lay press are addressing: our lack of military preparedness from the overweight/obesity epidemic.

The rise of ultra-processed food, the ultimate artificial food, is relevant to both the micro *and* macro damage incurred because of our exposure to it and its very production. I think many of you will agree after reading this book that these are serious issues needing to be addressed, sooner than later.

# PART 1

## The Addiction

"Quitting smoking is easy. I've done it a hundred times." Mark Twain, American author

I ask that you think of someone's daily routine, perhaps a friend, family member or coworker. Suppose for a moment that you, "Kate," are a busy single mother of three children, who has just gotten them off to school. By the time you get to work, you hadn't had enough time to get yourself breakfast or to pack a lunch, so you decide to go to the nearby coffee shop to grab a bite to get you going. Your stomach is growling and the ghrelin in your brain, the hormone that tells you that you are hungry, is signaling that you need to satisfy your stomach and your taste buds, and to do it so as quickly as possible. Mindful that you have an important meeting with your staff in 30 minutes, you order yourself a 24-ounce pumpkin spice latte (the calendar says it's coming up on Thanksgiving), an iced scone, and two bacon, cheese and egg sandwiches made with a white flour English muffin, and a brownie to satisfy your post-lunch sweet tooth.

You gulp the coffee and shove the scone in your mouth as you read your emails and check Instagram to see what your friends and some strangers are up to. It takes you all of ten minutes to finish your breakfast, as you head onto the building and throw your coat and backpack in your office. You head over to the conference room and meet your colleagues for the presentation you prepared for the upcoming ad campaign. On the conference table sits a few boxes of donuts, a few large muffins and assorted fruit. They all sit in front of the coffee pot and hot water for tea.

After a meeting that ran over the allotted time, replete with verbose co-workers and computer glitches, you head to your office to review emails. Your stomach is growling again and you have the beginnings of a headache.

You head to the vending machine and get yourself a bag of potato chips to hold you steady until lunch. The chips are gone by the time you hit your desk when a job applicant comes in to have her one-hour interview. After that's done you eat your lunch at your desk, and wash it down with a sweetened iced tea from the office fridge. Wiping the crumbs from the bacon, egg, and cheese sandwiches from your desk you stare at the chocolate brownie in front of you. Was that a flash of guilt you just felt? "I should have brought something healthier to have as a dessert," you say to yourself, considering that your doctor had told you the week prior at your yearly physical that you could stand to lose thirty pounds and that your hemoglobin A1C, a measure of your average blood glucose over the past three months, is too high and indicates that you are now prediabetic.

You cut the brownie in half and, congratulating yourself, wrap the uneaten half in plastic wrap and put it away. You eat the remaining portion of the brownie and go on with your day.

Your ex-husband is picking up the kids from school and has the kids for the weekend. Wrapping up your day at 5:30, you wonder whether you will have time to hit the gym before a 7:30 dinner you had arranged with a friend. Traffic is heavy as you make your way home and it's already a little past 6 when you start to change into your workout clothes. Just then your phone rings and it's your mother, who proceeds to tell you about the fight she had with your sister. Sitting down to console your mom, you absently eat a few pretzels that the kids had left out on the kitchen table. By the time the conversation ends, it's already closing in on 6:35 and the window of time to get to the gym has closed.

Shedding your workout clothes, you take a quick shower and wriggle into your dinner clothes. "Damn these pants are getting tight," you say to yourself as you look in the mirror. The Uber driver deposits you at the restaurant where your friend texts that she is running late. The waiter asks you if you would like a drink and, taking that microsecond to remind yourself that you just got a 15 percent salary increase and that your day has been stressful, you order an appletini with a sugar rim. With the tip, it's 20 USD.

Your cocktail is now half gone, your friend arrives and after greetings and small talk, you both peruse the menu. Your friend orders a salad and the chicken piccata, and you get your favorite, garlic bruschetta to start and pasta with clams in a white sauce. You ask your friend if she wants wine, which she does, and you both agree to a bottle instead of two glasses, reasoning you can flip a coin, the winner taking home the rest of the bottle.

The appetizers and the wine come and everything tastes so damned good. The wine is flowing as your tell yourself "Only one glass max tonight," but when the main courses come and the apple-tini and wine have taken their desired effect, you are enjoying the food and companionship so much that your hardly notice that the bottle is almost empty. "Little sense taking it home," you reason, so you and your friend drain the bottle. As the waiter takes the dishes away from the table, he asks if you have "saved room for dessert." Your companion demurs but you are craving your favorite after dinner treat on the menu, the cherry cheesecake. You think about what your doctor had said and feel the tug of your pants around your waist and, with some degree of pride, tell the waiter, "Just the check, please."

You are home by 9:45 but too wired to go to bed. You change into pajamas and settle yourself in front of the television, a small glass of Italian brandy in your hand. You watch a show on Amazon Prime until 11 and head upstairs to bed. After checking Facebook, Instagram, and a dating app in your bed, you put the phone aside and try to get some sleep, which does not come quickly or easily.

Now please imagine you are a 35-year-old unmarried trucker named Ted, living in rural Pennsylvania. You are a six-foot tall veteran and now drive a truck, where you spend most of your days and some of your nights on the road. In high school you wrestled at a weight of 155 pounds and by the time you left the army when you were 24, you weighed pretty much the same. But ever since you started trucking when you left the service you have packed on the pounds, so much so that you now weigh about 260 pounds. At the local diner breakfast consists of three eggs with cheese, three pieces of white toast with butter, orange juice, coffee and five strips of bacon. A snack on the road is a 24-ounce soda and a bag of fried pork rinds. Lunch is typically a double cheeseburger with fries, another large soda, and a processed single-serve apple pie for dessert. Your afternoon snack is another soda, potato chips and beef jerky. If you get home late that night you drop a 24-inch meat-lover's frozen pizza in the oven and enjoy the entire thing with a couple of beers in front of the TV. On the weekend, you look forward to going to the local all-you-can-eat buffet, where the owners always regret seeing you because they know they will be losing money when you walk through the door.

You haven't seen a doctor in years, but if you did, you'd be told you have high blood pressure, type 2 diabetes, and the beginnings of gout-related arthritis. You don't like going to doctors because you are afraid of what they might tell you, and the fact that they are going to make you get on a scale. You can't understand why you urinate so frequently and are so thirsty all the time (from your high blood sugar), and your right great toe is so red and sore (from your gout). When standing naked and looking down, you haven't seen your private parts in years.

If these visions of daily life seem familiar, you are not alone. From a dietary standpoint, they represent typical patterns for normal working people.

### What happened to Kate and Ted?

Kate's and Ted's dietary patterns are those of a hijacked and *inflamed* hypothalamus. The highly refined carbohydrates and the excessive amounts of saturated fat in what they have chronically ingested has altered their brains and disrupted the normal ghrelin (hunger)/ leptin (satiety and sense of fullness) balance. Their cravings represent exactly what Dr. Aronne alluded to in the *Forbes* article. "It's like your gas gauge points to empty all the time, whether or not the tank is full." And here we see it in real time. The "food" described here, full of exactly the *wrong* things to eat for a healthy body and brain, has been marketed, focus-group tested, concocted, and chemically engineered to hook its users to want more of it – in large quantities. Instead of eating health-inducing whole grain carbohydrates, fruits and vegetables that are high in dark, rich colors (and therefore rich in antioxidants), and other foods dense with fiber (which causes a slow rise in blood glucose and a gradual, tempered, and appropriate release of blood insulin), Kate is caught in a web of weight gain, prediabetes, possibly hypertension, and a host of other medical maladies. Ted is already there. As I stated in my 2021 book *What Your Doctor Won't Tell You* (Humanix), obesity truly is, in many ways, "the mother of all diseases."

Kate and Ted are victims whose hypothalamic activity has been biochemically *hijacked*. Like most of us, they have been bombarded since their early years by the advertising industry to eat this way. They have seen and heard untold numbers of ads peddling processed and mass-produced sugary cereals, chips, frozen pizzas, cookies, candies, ice cream, soft drinks, and, perhaps most importantly, fast food offered by the chain restaurants we all know. These products, most of which have large numbers of ingredients you need a degree in chemistry to understand and created in food laboratories, are synthesized for their taste, their texture, their mouth appeal, and their ability to get people to *crave* it and want more of it. The food industry knows this "bliss point," as some have called it.

The science of addiction is complex and has fostered a large field of scientific inquiry. There are many definitions of addiction, but the one from *Webster's Dictionary* is perhaps the most simple and clear:

"A compulsive, chronic, physiological or psychological need for a habit-forming substance, behavior, or activity, having harmful physical, psychological, or social effects and typically causing well-defined symptoms (such as irritability, tremors, or nausea) upon withdrawal or abstinence."

Traditionally, when one thinks of addiction or addicts, unfortunate judgmental and misguided images of intravenous drug abusers or skid-row winos come to mind. This has changed over the years to a degree, due primarily to the evolution of addictionology as a true medical science, whereby the victim of the condition is viewed as a sufferer of *disease* rather than someone who is morally bankrupt.

Like it or not, higher BMI persons are frequently viewed with disdain; it is thought that to at least some degree, the afflicted are responsible for their excessive weight. While it has been proven by evidenced-based science that maintaining a BMI at 25 or under is largely, but not always, associated with good health, the degree to which this is a matter of personal choice and genetics versus addiction appears to be more controversial.

And it is addiction itself that has led us to where we are. Addictions, by definition, always involve the central nervous system and the incredibly complex underlying biochemistry and physiology to which it is subject. Author and physician Gabor Mate, in his book *In the Realm of Hungry Ghosts*, has characterized addiction as "any repeated behavior, substance-related or not, in which a person feels compelled to persist, regardless of the negative impact on his life and the life of others." He also notes the four hallmarks of addiction, which in essence are compulsive engagement and pre-occupation with a behavior, inadequate control over the behavior, continuing the behavior or relapsing despite the harm it causes, and discomfort and irritability when the craved object is not available.

I think today's weight problem due to poor diets qualify here as an addiction.

Whereas the more commonly recognized addictions (illicit drugs, cigarettes, caffeine, alcohol, and so on) depend upon the actions of the neurotransmitter dopamine and a few others, the main players in the physiology of hunger – and its flipside, satiety – are ghrelin and leptin. It the most basic terms, ghrelin tells your brain that you are hungry, and leptin that you are full and have had enough to eat. It is much more complicated than that, of course, but that's the starting point to our discussion.

But to really understand the full story it is essential to under-stand the anatomy and physiology of the brain and central nervous system. This system is very much a hierarchical system and, without getting too technical, is based on anatomy (the hardware) and physiology (the operating system), working in concert to make the body "run." It's also akin to form and function. The central nervous system is generally more complex anatomically as evolution has revealed. The brain of *homo sapiens* is infinitely more complex than that of an earthworm, triceratops, or lizard. Let's look at the central nervous system before we speak of addiction in depth.

From bottom to top, from least evolved to most, the central nervous system (CNS) consists of the spinal cord, the medulla, the pons, the cerebellum, the midbrain, the diencephalon, and the cerebral hemispheres with their cortexes. The hypothalamus, where so many of our bodily functions are choreographed, resides between the two cerebral hemispheres, where it is part of the diencephalon. The thalamus also lives there.

Your hypothalamus is like the nervous system's Grand Central Station and is responsible for maintaining the body's "set points" (homeostasis) on many levels. Through your autonomic nervous system (both sympathetic and parasympathetic) and the transmission of neurotransmitters, coupled with the sending of important hormones to different parts of the body, the hypothalamus regulates body temperature, mood, sleep, sexual drive, hunger, thirst, blood pressure, and respiration. Because of its dual role in neurotransmission and hormonal regulation, it is the true link between the body's nervous and glandular systems. It straddles, therefore, three important disciplines in medicine: neurology, psychiatry, and endocrinology.

The hypothalamus receives signals from higher brain centers, like the cerebral cortex, and sends signals to other structures, like the pituitary gland. When it is diseased or damaged (say by trauma) the body's normal homeostasis can be disrupted and illness can occur. For our discussion on overweight/obesity and the role of the damaged hypothalamus, we will concentrate our attention there.

First there are ghrelin and leptin, the yin and yang of hunger homeostasis. Admittedly, the physiology of obesity is exceedingly complex. But since the focus of this book is overweight/ obesity due to hypothalamic inflammation and the brain's alteration due to UPF, I will restrict my discussion to that area of metabolic science. It has been known for many years that these two hormones exert a complementary effect with regard to your sense of hunger or fullness (satiety). Put simply, leptin puts the brakes on your hunger and tells you when you've had enough, and ghrelin tells you that you are hungry and to eat more. Drilling down further, science tells us that ghrelin:

- Has a lowering effect on insulin (the hormone lacking or completely absent in diabetics) sensitivity and secretion and is crucial in the synthesis and breakdown of both glucose (blood sugar) and glycogen (the stored form of glucose in the liver and skeletal muscle).

- Lowers the activity of the sympathetic nervous system.

- Reduces body heat production.

- Can even have a role in cancer and bone growth.

After a healthy person has had adequate food intake, leptin steps in to put the brakes on ghrelin's action, thereby telling the person to stop eating until food is needed once more for the needs of the body. For both Kate and Ted, that normal physiologic response has been altered.

This is where the scientists at Liverpool, Dr. Aronne, and many other researchers come in. A paper published in the February 2013 edition of *British Journal of Nutrition* elucidated the science of hypothalamic inflammation and the damage done to the ghrelin/leptin balancing act. Once again, from the *Forbes* article:

> "Over time, consuming too many calories from fat and simple sugars damages the nerves that conduct signals through the hypothalamus, affecting the function of leptin and ghrelin, and thus the body's ability to regulate weight and metabolism, says Aronne. 'Because of this damage, the signals don't get through about how much fat is stored.'"

A few years later, a paper published in the *Annual Review of Physiology* in 2015 by Martin Valdearcos, Allison W. Xu, and Suneil K. Koliwad of the University of California, San Francisco's Department of Medicine and Diabetes Center revealed additional related findings. They observed:

> "... hypothalamic inflammation induced by dietary excess precedes the onset of overt obesity and occurs much earlier than inflammation or metabolic disturbances in peripheral tissue. This primacy suggests that hypothalamic inflammation plays an acute role in modulating normal metabolic physiology and is an early driver of the pathophysiology associated with overnutrition ... This hypothalamic circuit of energy balance is amenable to feedback regulation by circulating metabolic signals, including those from nutritional hormones such as leptin and insulin ... The specificity of dietary saturated fatty acids as inducers of inflammation within the MBH (a section of the hypothalamus) has been assessed in several ways."

The investigators went on to say that when saturated fatty acids were introduced into the study mice's system – whether by feeding, introduction in the bloodstream, or directly into the central system – hypothalamic inflammation and dysfunction resulted. Conversely, these injuries subsequently improved (evidenced by "lowered inflammatory responses and with the restoration of leptin and insulin sensitivity") when the diet was favorably altered, commenting that "dietary induced obesity in mice is partially reversed when saturated fats are replaced by unsaturated fats."

Desiring further evidence of the link between bad food/ultra processed food and hypothalamic inflammation/obesity, I searched for more contemporary evidence. I find an abundance. In research medical centers and universities as far flung and disparate as the United Kingdom, South Africa, Germany, and here at home at Yale University, scientists were busy refining the complex biochemical and physiologic mechanisms of this toxic association. Indeed, Professor of Cellular and Molecular Physiology Sabrina Diano at Yale University School of Medicine weighed in as well, and blamed diets with high saturated fat content and carbohydrates for hypothalamic inflammation and the resultant dysfunction caused by obesity and malnutrition. So did many others.

I had seen enough. The evidence, as nuanced and complex as it was, was clear. An image popped into my head. It was that of a black and white, old-time movie, featuring a paperboy hawking newspapers on the street corner. He shouts *"EXTRA, EXTRA, READ ALL ABOUT IT! HUNGER HACKS HYPOTHALAMUS, HORMONES GO HAYWIRE!"*

Recall earlier what Dr. Mate had to say about addiction, where dopamine plays an important part. Regarding overeating, older research strongly implicates activation of endogenous opioids (endorphins), as well as a surge of dopamine when fatty, sweet and/or salty food is ingested, in weight gain. This made me wonder if there was a potential fit here between the ghrelin/leptin inflammatory model, dopamine, and other clinical conditions. Sure, enough studies have found correlations between a high UPF diet and systemic (meaning within the entire body itself) inflammatory influences on the brain. (Bad diets seem to correlate as well with low dopamine in a subset of depression and with low dopamine receptors in obesity as well. An *Emory News Center* report of January

26, 2023, quoted a study recently that found that levodopa, a drug that heightens dopamine in the brain, may be able to "reverse brain reward circuitry, ultimately improving symptoms of depression.") And a *Science News* report in April of 2021 written by Roger Adan, PhD of University Medical Center Utrecht in the Netherlands revealed that there is ". . . communication between fat storages (via a hormone called leptin) and the brain's dopamine reward system. This leptin-dopamine axis is critically important for body weight control, but its modes of action were not well understood."

So, if hypothalamic inflammation and its subsequent damage from processed food impairs the normal activity of the "fullness" hormone leptin, does this disrupt the crucial leptin-dopamine relationship as well? Much more research is needed, but a deeper understanding of the biochemical interactions of ghrelin, leptin, dopamine and other neurotransmitters and hormones may tailor future therapies in not only obesity and depression, but other pathologies as well.

Leaving this alchemy aside, let's return to Kate, whose diet and lifestyle belie the appearance of much of the trouble we see today with regards to both physical, mental, and even emotional health. Kate is a busy and successful (at least in the eyes of society) professional with many challenges. She is strapped for time, has an abysmal diet and has not taken her doctor's advice to heart. She displays several behavioral and physical features that put her at risk for other diseases: her body mass index is high, she suffers from time urgency, her Hemoglobin A1C is high, and she tipples the alcohol a fair amount. She is also under stress and uses her electronics in bed.

Let's look at her daily food intake. It is dominated by saturated fat, refined carbohydrates, sugar, and displays a lack of fiber. Her breakfast was a large pumpkin spiced latte (sugar and fat) and an iced scone (more sugar and fat). The potato chips for her morning snack (more ultra processed saturated fat and refined carbohydrates) and her lunch of bacon, egg, and cheese sandwiches (more of the same) add more inflammation to her already on-fire body and impaired hypothalamus. The *coup de gras* comes at dinner, with the appletini with sugar rim, the bruschetta (more white starch), the wine (sugar, sugar, sugar) and the perhaps the pasta (depending on the type).

Oh, and the half brownie after lunch.

If you think this representation of a typical daily diet is unrealistic, I respectfully disagree, for it has been estimated that about 70 percent of the American diet is UPF. Tragically, this diet represents the way most people eat in this country. Actually, I'm wrong; this diet is probably *better* than what most people eat in this country. I left out the processed cereal, donuts, instant oatmeal, subs, hot dogs, hamburgers, pizza, white bread, white rice, soft drinks, chips, cookies, cakes, pies, and other confections most people have before they even get to dinner. And then there's dinner. Heat-and-serve entrees, take-out Mexican, take-out Chinese, take-out anything in heavy sauces, sausage, thick crust frozen pizza, beer, wine, liquor, and soda. Then pick your dessert. All likely to be highly processed and highly unhealthy.

In a country where the national meal is a hamburger, fries, and a milk shake, or you can order an abomination like fried chicken and waffles at a restaurant, must we wonder why our brains are so inflamed, why we are addicted, why 70 percent of us are overweight or obese?

And what exactly is this UPF? In his 2023 book *Ultra-Processed PEOPLE, The Science Behind Food That Isn't Food*, physician

Chris Van Tulleken argues that it is UPF that is the primary cause of myriad health issues we see today. He quotes one accepted definition of UPF:

"Formulations of ingredients, mostly of exclusive industrial use, made by a series of industrial processes, many requiring sophisticated equipment and technology ... Processes and ingredients used to manufacture ultra-processed foods are designed to create highly profitable (low-cost ingredients, long shelf life, emphatic branding) convenient (ready-to-consume) hyper-palatable products liable to displace freshly prepared dishes ..."

Isn't *that* a mouthful!

Back to Kate, who does not even know what she does not know. And why should she? She didn't go to medical school. She's not a nutritionist. She's just a typical American, brought up in America, watching American TV, listening to American radio, and going out to American parties and social events. She wouldn't know ghrelin from her father's AMC Gremlin. If asked where her hypothalamus was located, she might know its somewhere in her head but she wouldn't have a clue as to what it does. Her diet is replete with some of the worst ingredients her body, and especially her brain, can take. And her time-stressed doctor, who has given her the boilerplate 15-second "exercise more and eat more fruits and vegetables" routine has been of little help to her.

Her diet, day after day, month after month and year after year, has wreaked havoc on her hypothalamus. Her country song for her state of health might go "my leptin ain't workin' and my ghrelin's gone berserkin'", all thanks to an inflamed body and hypothalamus. And the bad news is that some of that is irreversible. Some of it – not all.

But for Ted, the symptoms, signs, and prognosis are more ominous. He already has hypertension and diabetes, likely due to his horrific diet and sedentary job. If he does not change his ways, he is advancing to a life of chronic disease and early death. But it will take herculean effort for him to beat his bad food addiction and save himself, likely due to health illiteracy, habit, and certainly addiction.

Crucial to the understanding of how truly destructive Kate's and Ted's eating habits are, it is important to tease out definitions of the major players in this drama: body mass index, glycemic index, glycemic load, saturated fat, refined carbohydrates, oxidative stress, and neurotransmitters, hormones, and cytokines.

*Body mass index*, or BMI, is defined as a person's weight in kilograms divided by the square of his or her height in meters. "Healthy" BMI is considered to be between 18.5 and 24.9. It is only a very rough indicator of health and is an imperfect index regarding disease states. There are normal BMI ill people and above normal BMI healthy people.

*Glycemic index*, or GI, is a measure of how rapidly certain foods can make your blood sugar rise. Low GI foods have an index of 55 and lower. High GI foods have an index of 70 and greater. Moderate GI is between 56 and 69. The related term *glycemic load*, or GL, represents how much the ingested food will increase a person's serum glucose level after eating. A formula that links the two is: grams of carbohydrate in a food x GI divided by 100 = GL. A GL is said to be high if it exceeds 20, 11 to 19 is medium, and less than 10 is low. Of note is that studies have linked a lower GI and GI diet to a reduced risk of developing type 2 diabetes.

*Saturated fats* are those whose fatty acid chains have single chemical bonds, like those derived from animal fats. In contrast, plant-derived and fish-sourced fats are mostly not saturated fats. A diet heavy in saturated fat can put a person at increased risk for cancer, cardiovascular disease (heart attack, stroke, peripheral vascular disease), and diabetes.

When we speak of *refined carbohydrates*, we mean those carbohydrates derived from sugars, like table sugar, high fructose corn syrup, and other sugars found in processed foods, as well as grains that have had their fiber and more nutritious elements (like vitamins and minerals) removed, or stripped away. These types of carbohydrates, when ingested in sufficient amounts over time, can place a person at risk for similar diseases as a diet rich in saturated fats. Refined carbohydrates found in processed food tend to carry a high GI and GL.

*Oxidative stress* is a sophisticated physiological concept that may carry profound implication in human diseases, such as diabetes, cancer, cardiovascular disease, and other disorders. Simply put it refers to an abnormal relationship between production and buildup of reactive oxygen species, forms of oxygen molecules that are produced as byproducts of metabolism, and antioxidants. These forms, like hydrogen peroxide, superoxide, and others can harm cellular elements that ensure proper cellular function and integrity. It is a growing area of research regarding human disease states.

A *neurotransmitter* is a chemical messenger released by nerves to other nerves or tissues in the body in order to affect a certain function or physiologic response. The four neurotransmitters most well-known are acetylcholine, dopamine, serotonin, and glutamate. Adrenaline (epinephrine), gamma aminobutyric acid (GABA) and oxytocin are also neurotransmitters, each with specific functions. Some of them play a role in appetite regulation.

*Hormones* are also chemical messengers released by the endo-crine glands, like the thyroid gland, pituitary, pancreas, and adrenal glands, that are involved in specific bodily functions. The islet cells of the pancreas, for example, makes the insulin we use to regulate blood sugar, among other things. Type 1 diabetes occurs when the pancreas cannot make enough or, for that matter, any insulin to maintain adequate blood sugar balance. Type 2 diabetes usually occurs later in life than type 1 and is characterized by a relative lack of insulin production or a resistance to the insulin you already are making.

*Cytokines* are protein molecules that play a central role in immunity, inflammation, and autoimmune disease (where the body attacks its own tissues) and are significant for their ability to tell other cells within the bloodstream how to fight infectious agents and other intruders. These proteins gained a prominent reputation during the Covid-19 pandemic with the term "cytokine storm" for their potential in causing serious total body inflammatory states.

I have defined these players in more detail to illustrate what is going on in Kate's, Ted's and many people's bodies due to diets rich in saturated fat, refined carbohydrates, sugars and UPF. *Please bear in mind that there are many interrelated and overlapping processes going on in our discussion of the deleterious health effects of high body mass index and processed food – especially regarding inflammation, oxidative stress, and cytokines – that are beyond the scope of this book.* But they are important to mention for the sake of completeness and integrity and I encourage you, if you are so inclined and/or have a background in the biological sciences, to do more research yourself. Also know that I will be quoting a healthy body of scientific research directly, not because I can't explain it myself, but because oftentimes the words of the researchers themselves carry more weight. Please bear with these many references if you feel they are much to process.

Returning to Kate's diet, the sugary and fatty latte, the glazed, white flour scone and the bacon, egg, and cheese sandwiches, so rich with refined flour and saturated fat, are exactly the wrong things to eat to foster good health. Studies confirm that diets rich in these foods place Kate at risk for the diseases I mentioned above, and she is well on her way to type 2 diabetes as evidenced by her elevated hemoglobin A1C. All through the day the foods she eats, so deficient in the glucose and insulin-modulating effect of high fiber consumption, is causing her body to react in sugar highs and plummeting crashes. Her diet is rich with high GI and GL ingredients, causing rapid rises in her blood sugar and causing a surge of insulin from her pancreas to bring the sugar levels down in her bloodstream. This taxes the pancreas which must – over a lifetime – manufacture the insulin we need to maintain metabolic balance.

The ravages to Kate's brain and body continue with the half brownie, the cocktail (made with a sugary, premixed apple flavored syrup), the white bread bruschetta, and the wine. The only low GI food is the pasta, whose GI of 55 makes it the winner for lowest GI and GL food of the day. Ted's diet is even worse and he has the diseases to show for it. Incredibly, it is exactly how so many of us eat today. Horrifying.

As we will see in part IV of this book, there are so many dietary substitutions both Kate and Ted could make to spare their bodies the systemic and localized inflammatory onslaught they unleash every day. This *insult* to their anatomy and physiology goes on without their knowledge. I'm sure if they truly knew what they were doing to themselves and what paths they were leading themselves down, they might take serious steps to change their diet and thus their lives. For what Kate and Ted are doing enhances not only their risk for developing the biggest causes of morbidity (illness) and mortality (death) in the United States (cardiovascular disease) but is taxing our economy with the money we all must spend to care for her present and future medical issues.

And an *insult* it is, for that's how physicians describe, literally, any damage – whether behavioral or by actual physical trauma – to a patient's anatomy or physiology. These *assaults* on the system come in many forms, the most prominent of which (when speaking of our diets) are:

- the cardiovascular system, particularly the heart, blood vessels, large, small, and in between
- the endocrine or "glandular" system, particularly with reference to the pancreas
- the central and peripheral nervous systems, especially the hypothalamus
- the joints and musculoskeletal system, from the increased stress that a high BMI puts on them
- our sleep quality, with special reference to obstructive sleep apnea (OSA)
- the adipose tissue, which is actually an organ in itself
- the gastrointestinal system and the bacteria that inhabit it

- kidney function

- our liver, in the form of a rising problem, non-alcoholic fatty liver disease, or NAFLD

- our immune systems and our ability to prevent cancer and fight infection

- our rheumatologic systems, with regard to generalized inflammation in the body

- our psyches, which are affected by depression, anxiety, and other emotional maladies

I hope you are beginning to see why the subject of this book has far-reaching relevance for so many of us.

In my 2021 book *What Your Doctor Won't Tell You: The Real Reasons You Don't Feel Good and What You Can Do About It*, I listed the major causes of morbidity and mortality in the US. In that book I quoted an article from the October 24, 2018 issue of *USA Today*, written by Kate Morgan. In that article, the top 5 medical afflictions in the US were:

1. high blood pressure

2. major depression

3. high blood cholesterol

4. coronary artery disease

5. Type 2 diabetes.

That same year, the CDC's mortality data, as well as some key related data reported by authors Jiaquan Xu, MD, Sherry Murphy, BS, Kenneth Kochanek, MA and Elizabeth Arias, PhD, revealed the leading causes of death:

1. heart disease

2. cancer

3. unintentional injuries

4. chronic lower respiratory diseases

5. stroke

I hope you see a pattern here. Cardiovascular disease (heart attack, stroke, and so on), cancer, and metabolic disease (diabetes) figure prominently. We can only conjecture the impact her eating habits are having on Kate and Ted, but let's take it one step further. Listen to what Dr. Tulleken had to say when he put himself on a diet of UPF:

"When I went back for testing at UCL (University College London) at the end of the diet, the results were spectacular. I had gained 6 kg. (about 13.2 pounds) . . . Additionally, my appetite hormones were totally deranged. The hormone that signals fullness barely responded to a large meal, while the hunger hormone was sky high just moments after eating. There was a five-fold increase in leptin . . . while my levels of C-reactive protein, a marker that indicates inflammation, had doubled."

He went on to say that there were changes in his brain MRI scan, which he called "terrifying." Admitting that the results of his scan were hard to interpret, he concluded it may represent "a tussle between parts of my brain wanting the food more or less subconsciously and the parts that consciously understood the harms."

Later in that same chapter he was quick to note that "UPF is consistently associated with higher scores on food addiction scales compared to real food."

We've discussed the impact on health of foods that are high in sugar, saturated fat, and refined carbohydrates, as well as the addictive potential of both UPF and diets rich in these substances. I've presented a typical daily American diet to show you how damaging, nutrient-poor, and inflammatory our eating habits have become. All of this puts us at increased risk for overweight/obesity, and some of the top causes of morbidity and mortality. We've discussed some basic terminology to gain a better understanding of how all this works out anatomically and physiologically. Let's look at the backstory of how we got here, and who benefits from it.

# PART 2

## The Background **and Who Benefits**

"For the love of money is the root of all evil . . ."
1 Timothy 6:10 King James Version

The story of processed food is as old as human civilization itself. If we roughly define processed food as any ingested matter that is altered from its original state, then a hunk of cow muscle cooked on a fire, table salt, bread, and the juice of an orange or apple all technically qualify as processed food. Evelyn Kim, writing in 2013 in *Scientific American*, traced some familiar and not so familiar milestones in processed food. From oldest to more contemporary, she summarized her findings:

- roasted meat, 1.8 million years ago
- bread, 30,000 years ago
- beer, 7000 BC

- tortillas, 6700 BC
- wine, 5400 BC
- cheese, 5000 BC
- olive oil, 4500 BC
- palm oil, 3000 BC
- pickles, 2400 BC
- noodles, 2000 BC
- chocolate, 1900 BC
- bacon, 1500 BC
- jiang (a flavoring often found in miso and soy sauce), 1000 BC
- sugar, 500 BC
- mustard, 400 BC
- kimchi, 700 AD
- sushi, 700 AD
- tofu, 965 AD
- salt cod, 10th century
- peanut butter, 15th century
- coffee, mid-15th century
- carbonated water, 1767
- corn flakes, 1894
- MSG, 1908
- SPAM, 1926
- chicken nuggets, 1950s
- high fructose corn syrup, 1957
- Tang, 1959
- lab-grown meat, 2013

It is interesting to see how many of these items are currently part of our diets in one way or another. The evolution of what we eat and why we eat it *in that form* is a fascinating topic, one that has been covered in detail by many authors. But behind every processed food story there lies a reason for its development and popularity. Beer and wine made their users feel initially elated and then drunk if the imbibing continued. SPAM developed as a cheap and practical way to feed armies. Coffee was not only a stimulant but served as a medicine of sorts for lassitude and other maladies. It also fostered a sophisticated social phenomenon, particularly with regard to coffee houses. (My favorite composer, Johann Sebastian Bach, even wrote a Coffee Cantata, where a father scolds his daughter for her coffee addiction.) And of course, many people interested in making money saw opportunity in processing food.

Today the sale of processed foods is a multi-*trillion*-dollar industry. According to Statista.com, worldwide revenue from the food market itself is expected to reach 12.97 trillion dollars in 2028, much of it related to processed food. Regarding food overall, the year 2023 found the tenth consecutive year of increasing global food revenue, and the projections are that this trend will continue.

The rapid ascent of processed food mirrored the rise in other technologies. The older methods of food processing – salting, drying, fermentation, pickling, and canning – have gradually given way to more current and sophisticated ways of preserving and altering what we eat. Refrigeration and freezing, the use of an increasing number of preservatives, food irradiation and high-pressure treatment of edibles as well as surface cleansing became more common. There are advanced technologies that I as a physician and student of the sciences have difficulty comprehending, such as cold plasma and pulsed electric fields. All these methods, both old and new, have enabled producers to satisfy the ever-increasing needs of their customer base with regard to sanitation, convenience, taste, "mouthfeel," and importantly, cost. Cost, as we will see later, is a primary driver behind UPF consumption because so many calories – health-wrecking as they are – for so cheap a price have never been more available. The myriad companies involved in processed food creation saw dollar signs. And as the numbers indicate they were richly rewarded for their efforts.

Growing up, like all the kids I knew and people all over our country and in so many parts of the developed world, I was an unwitting victim of those efforts. Even my physician father was oblivious (he was to develop type 2 diabetes by his mid-forties).

When I look back on my own childhood in the late 1950s and through the 1960s and early part of the 1970s, I shudder now to consider what I thought was of as an ordinary diet. And of course, I thought it was normal. How could I have possibly known any differently? I was inundated with ads on television while watching Bugs Bunny, I Love Lucy or The Dick Van Dyke Show for everything from Kellogg's Frosted Flakes to Hostess Ho-Ho's to Tastykake cake and pies. My experience as an American child of those times is something with which many of my readers can identify. Always a squeamish eater, I existed on a staple of sugary cereals, stove-top popcorn, peanut butter sandwiches made with white bread, ice cream sandwiches, sugary sodas, hot dogs, TV dinners, Nestles Quik and Hershey's Chocolate Syrup in whole milk, and God knows what else. In many ways it's a miracle I'm still alive.

By the time I was 16 years old and playing football for my school team, I was tipping the scales at nearly 200 pounds. A meal for myself that late summer after two-a-day football practice was a half-liter of Coca Cola and a Domino's pizza. Dessert was some Sara Lee pound cake or banana cake. I still don't recall eating a piece of fruit or some leafy greens.

In 1972 I transitioned from pediatric care to a doctor who treated adults. The doctor I began to see was a friend of my father's. (By sheer chance I happened to treat him years later when he was 96 years old and I was 57, but that's another story). He ran some blood tests and told me that my blood lipids were badly deranged. My cholesterol was too high and my "bad" cholesterol, LDL, way elevated as well. He also told me that I weighed too much and – as a sibling and a son of people who had diabetes (my sister with type

1 and my father with type 2) – he cautioned me that I had better change my ways.

His warning worked. I stopped drinking soda altogether and added more fruits and vegetables to my diet. I lost about 20 pounds and my blood lipid tests returned to the normal range.

It was too bad I didn't fully heed his advice, for when I went off to college in September of 1976 at Emory University (the "Coca Cola" school, as evidenced by the institution's historical relationship to the soft drink giant and the 100 million dollar grant it received from Coca Cola in 1979), I was back to eating poison. Hamburgers, French fries, mass produced pizza, milk shakes, sub sandwiches made with processed meat and white flour – and worse. I was so caught up in the pre-med circus I didn't have time or the proclivity to think differently. I still cannot recall eating a piece of fruit or a salad.

By the time I entered medical school in Boston in the fall of 1979 not much had changed. I almost never cooked for myself, and most of my food intake came from convenience stores, chain fast food restaurants, the hospital cafeteria and whatever I could chisel off my roommate. Astounding is the fact that I recall receiving virtual no teaching in medical school on nutrition and healthy eating. Sure, I studied biochemistry, with its dry lectures on the Krebs citric acid cycle, the synthesis of proteins, fats and carbohydrates, and the all-important production of ATP to keep the body running. But there was absolutely no discussion of the dangers of bad food or UPF. Ultra processed food wasn't even a concept back then.

My internal medicine internship in Baltimore was no different, and anesthesiology residency in Miami was much the same. I remember the on-call attending anesthesiologist would buy us cash-strapped residents soda and pizza to keep us going through the night. Morning conferences *always* offered the same thing: coffee and donuts, donuts and still more donuts. We used to jokingly refer to the morbidity and mortality meeting every Wednesday morning as "Death and Donuts."

By the time I became an attending physician myself I weighed close to 200 pounds and stood 5 feet 10 inches, for a BMI of about 28.7, the unhealthy range. It wasn't until the mid-1990s, when I was in my mid-thirties that I heard about a boot camp fitness program. I enrolled and it was the very first time I was taught to watch what I ate. I cut out the refined carbs and sugar and watched my saturated fat intake. I increased my consumption of fruit, vegetables, and water and although I still cheated occasionally, managed to lose about 35 pounds over a year or so. People who had not seen me for a long time wondered if I had some dreadful illness I was so gaunt. My old clothing hung from me.

At poker games with my dad and his contemporaries during the two terms Bill Clinton was in office as the US President, I looked around the table at a familiar scene. All the men there, in their forties to their late sixties, were overweight, on multiple medications (as evidenced by their discussions at the poker table with my dad) and ate horribly. Here were attorneys, mortgage brokers, businessmen, accountants – presumably educated, intelligent people – gorging themselves on processed sandwiches of nitrate-riddled, fatty deli meat, salty pickles, processed chips, soda, and cookies. It was a typical and sorry sight to take in.

Ever since then, these three decades later, I have maintained a weight of about 157 pounds, with a body mass index of between 22.5 and 24. My cholesterol has remained in the normal range despite having a family history of elevated blood lipids. Most of my contemporaries are on statins.

My story is unusual in one respect; I lost weight as I aged, not gained. Most of my friends at my high school reunions put on the pounds, as is the predictable pattern in America as we grow older. I'm not bragging about this, I'm just fortunate to have been enlightened. Enlightened and sensitized by watching my father and sister deal with their afflictions.

My life before my "enlightenment" is a clear reflection of the inherent dangers of our eating habits and our increasingly sedentary lifestyles (I refer to this later, in part III). It is a direct result of marketing, lust for profit and a determination to convert hordes of people into junk-addicted victims. Surely personal responsibility is responsible for part of the picture but the forces working against us are evidently too great for most people. Indeed, three quarters of us are now overweight or obese, an all-time high.

A perfect example of this appeared in *The Washington Post* on December 18, 2019, in an article by writer Laura Reiley entitled "Coca-Cola internal documents reveal efforts to sell to teens, despite obesity crisis." Noting that "obesity rates for children have tripled since the 1970s" and that "childhood obesity is estimated to cost 14 billion dollars annually in direct health expenses", the author quotes Gary Ruskin, co-director of a group called U. S. Right to Know, who warned against Coke's effort to portray, according to the article, sugary sodas as not so damaging to people's health:

> "One of these is Coca-Cola's efforts to evade responsibility for the global obesity epidemic ... Even though the health problems are quite severe in the U. S., we

live under *de facto* corporate control; the food industry is incredibly powerful in the U. S. What's insidious here is a health campaign that is using tobacco's tactics, promoting alternative science in a way that advances the notion that sugary sodas aren't really so bad ..."

She went on to quote Benjamin Wood, a then PhD candidate at Australia's Deakin University, and one of the authors of the study:

"We wanted to raise awareness of these hidden tactics and strategies to target teenagers and their mothers ... Coke also uses the recruitment of role models for young children."

Coca-Cola's story in gaining market share, especially among vulnerable populations, is representative of aggressive and disingenuous marketing efforts across the UPF industry spectrum. The Pan American Health Organization (PAHO) made some bold statements in their article "Marketing of Ultra-processed and Processed Food and Non-alcoholic Drink products." Their key points were that:

- UPF marketing fosters heavy consumption of sugar, saturated fat, trans fat, and salt. This fosters weight gain and the health problems that go along with that.
- Marketing regulation is needed to curb this effect.
- The regulation of this marketing is "feasible."

Despite these noble efforts, which came in May 2010 on the heels of the World Health Assembly's adopting of the World

Health Organization's Set of Recommendations on the "Marketing of Foods and Non-alcoholic Beverages to Children," we haven't seen much progress. In fact, the Center for Disease Control revealed in a February 2020 National Center for Health Statistics brief that from 1999-2000 up until 2017-2018, age adjusted obesity prevalence increased from 30.5 percent to 42.4 percent and severe obesity almost doubled from 4.7 percent to 9.2 percent.

So much for the well-meaning efforts of the PAHO and WHO.

If you want a more detailed discussion of the history behind the rise of processed food, I refer you to Dr. Chris van Tulleken's *Ultra-Processed PEOPLE: The Science Behind Food That Isn't Food*, Dr. David Kessler's *The End of Overeating: Taking Control of the American Appetite* and journalist and reporter Michael Moss's *Salt Sugar Fat: How the Food Giants Hooked Us*. Rather than rehashing their excellent work or quoting example after example of how the bad food industry tries to hook you, I think it more illuminating to let the people who actually study this topic as their life's work weigh in.

An article published in the January 26, 2021 issue of *Globalization and Health* by Benjamin Wood (the same Benjamin Wood from the *Washington Post* article above), Owain Williams, *et al*, entitled "Market strategies used by processed food manufacturers to increase and consolidate their power: a systemic review and document analysis" codified their findings in a damning indictment of the processed food industry. Referring to the role these companies play in "driving unhealthy diets, one of the leading contributors to the global burden of disease," the authors pull no punches.

Specifically, they cited companies' willingness to adopt "market-strategy dimension" (by augmenting brand value) and at the same time fostering "non-market strategy dimension" (via political and consumer legitimacy). While acknowledging the connection between unhealthy food and a sicker populace, the worldwide driving forces and institutional constructs that support their activities, and the use of political strategies to reach their goals (that is, "political donations, lobbying, and regulatory capture . . .") they identify six distinct "interconnected strategic objectives specific to dominant processed food manufacturers":

- cut competition with rivals and subdue smaller ones

- elevate the barriers to enter the market by new players

- neutralize "market disruptors and drive dietary displacement in favour of their products." (italics mine)

- raise their buying power "over suppliers."

- raise selling power "over retailers and distributors."

- "leverage informational power asymmetries in relations with consumers."

Of the six items above, I found the third and the sixth most disturbing. These actions, in my mind at least, represent *the* most reprehensible selling methods of the processed food giants: the actual exchange of health-fostering food with health-wrecking ingestibles, and a desire to "withhold, manipulate or use misleading process and product-related information on food labels . . . such as the use of deceptive health and nutrition claims, misleading marketing . . . and greenwashing."

Item six was just a fancy way of saying "lie to them."

These methods appear to be representative of the UPF industry, illustrated by what Michael Moss described in his book *Salt,*

*Sugar, Fat: How the Food Giants Hooked Us.* In that book he describes a Minneapolis meeting of the food giants in April of 1999, where representatives from Pillsbury (the host), Kraft, Nestle, Nabisco, General Mills, Coca-Cola, Mars, and other food giants met to discuss their industry and shared responsibility in creating health problems worldwide by making people fatter. There, Moss reveals "how they would respond to the evening's most delicate matter: the notion that they and their companies had played a central role in creating this health crisis." Also at the meeting was Michael Mudd, a vice president of the Kraft company. He warned the assembled food moguls, in a 114-slide presentation, about the health dangers of their collective products, particularly with regard to children and specifically in reference to "diabetes, heart disease, hypertension, gallbladder disease, osteoarthritis" and different forms of cancer, especially "breast, colon and that of the uterine lining . . ." Mudd admitted to what the executives have spent their careers achieving: "Ubiquity of inexpensive, good-tasting, super-sized, energy-dense food." It was a remarkable meeting in many ways.

Scientists, in particular a man named Howard Moskowitz, were instrumental in achieving the previously referenced "bliss point" for processed and ultra-processed foods. This concept relates to finding a perfect ingredient balance of sugar, salt, and fat, to achieve the maximum pleasure perception (sometimes referred to as "deliciousness"). The executives all knew about this concept and made sure that there were ongoing efforts at Kraft, Mars, Coca-Cola, and others to increase market share, satisfy shareholders and relentlessly outdo their competitors to achieve these objectives.

In many ways the morally questionable actions of these food processors should remind us of similar marketing tactics employed by the tobacco industry, alcohol producers, and the makers of opioid medications. (For example, we doctors were led by the nose into contributing to the opioid epidemic by not being skeptical enough when it came to opioid medication prescribing and guidelines some 25 years ago. Some research estimates reveal that in the United States alone in the 12-month period concluding on January 31, 2023 there were 109,600 overdose related deaths, or an average of 300 deaths *per day*, as compared to 841,000 from the *entire period* from 1999 to 2020.) And despite the efforts of people like Michael Mudd, who gave that presentation over 24 years ago, things have only deteriorated. People have heavier now, disease is more prevalent, and there appears to be no end in sight.

The food giants – whose names you see every day in your convenience store, gas stations, grocery shops, airports vendors, schools, train stations, and universities and are ever present on your TVs, social media, radio, billboards, and whatever form of popular culture you take in daily – continue to make huge profits and bear at least partial, if not the majority of, responsibility for the world's high BMI-related health fallout.

As I write these words there is an informative infographic created by Oxfam International that is making its way around the internet retitled "Terrifying Infographic Proves That Only 10 Companies Control Everything We Eat and Drink." It's a very busy graphic but if you focus on the main players and closely examine the subsidiary brands, you will recognize virtually every major label in the processed food and UPF universe. The major names listed are Nestle, PepsiCo, Coca-Cola, General Mills, Unilever, Kellogg's, Danone, Associated British Foods plc, Mars, and Mondelez International (formerly Kraft foods). These companies, confirmed by a *Knowledge Sourcing Intelligence* 2022 report ("Global Processed Food Market Size, Share, Opportunities, COVID-19 Impact, And

Trends By Processing Method, etc") on the global processed food market, form the core entities responsible for the trillions of dollars earned worldwide on the sale of their products. This report, 118 pages in length, touts the sales trajectory expected in the global market of these products, which is expected to go from 1.632 trillion USD in 2020 to 2.379 trillion USD in 2027. The authors of the original report take a rather dry, clinical approach in my view, and have clearly sold their souls to the devil when it comes to skirting the potential health effects of the products discussed. They say that "The rising demand for quick and conveniently available food . . . has primarily been caused by a relative reduction in the leisure hours available to individuals, causing them to switch to packaged food . . . the working-class population is getting busier in their corporate lives, frozen fruits and vegetables can stay fresher for longer and the sensitive vitamins and nutrients remain intact in the food."

Really? There's no mention of the untold number of other health-compromising ingredients, the salt, sugar, trans fat, and other saturated fats present in the product that scientists have proven again and again to be responsible for a global health crisis. They even have the audacity to mention that "Strict rules and guidelines must be followed during the processing of foods that reach consumers to ensure that no adverse effects occur and that the consumer's health does not deteriorate." Where is the punch line in that joke?

As impressive as the revenue and profits from the sale of these "foods" are, we have to look at the other major beneficiary of the global ubiquity of processed food and UPF – the pharmaceutical industry. Big Pharma is the clear winner when it comes to riding on the coattails of processed food makers, and the reasons should be clear. As the world's population grows in girth and body mass index, the concomitant diseases associated with this change in human anatomy and physiology become prime targets for drug makers. After all, somebody must be there to peddle the pills and inject-ables to treat the increase in diabetes, hypertension, degenerative joint disease, and autoimmune diseases caused by the ever-rising tide of bad food. According to a December 21, 2023 Statista.com report, published by Matej Mikulic, global pharmaceutical sales totaled 1.48 trillion dollars in 2022. They report meteoric growth projections for the next few years, saying that sales in 2026 should reach the following levels by region:

- North America: 774 billion

- European Union: 295 billion

- Southeast and East Asia: 267 billion

- China: 185 billion

- Latin America: 170 billion

- Europe non-EU, including UK: 82 billion

- Japan: 74 billion

- Indian subcontinent: 52 billion

- Commonwealth of Independent States: 40 billion

- Middle East: 29 billion

- Oceania: 19 billion

The cumulative sales for all the regions clearly will dwarf present levels if the projections are anywhere near accurate. And it should surprise no one that the rise in sales for pharmaceuticals occur in lockstep with the global obesity issue.

*IQVIA Institute* reports that total global sales for pharmaceuticals will reach 1.9 trillion USD by 2027 and issued a compelling expose on January 18, 2023 breaking down key factors in this growth. Here were some of the highlights of the report, a clear reflection of Big Pharma's windfall from deteriorating health globally:

- More people are using more medications. "Defined daily doses" grew by 36 percent in the past 10 years. They do admit that some of this growth has increased due to patient access. (I believe more ill people is the major cause.)
- Covid 19 has been a factor.
- There is growth related to specialty medicines, particularly in the areas of cancer therapy, immunology, rare neurological diseases, Alzheimer's disease, and migraine.

It is my opinion that our diets' propensity to increase the risks of some cancers, the risk of Alzheimer's and degenerative neurologic diseases (more on that in Part III) and worsening outcomes from Covid-19 infection in populations where there is an increase in BMI (I will discuss this later as well) reflect these projections.

*IQVIA* also issued a report entitled "The Global Use of Medicines" in January of 2023, where global spending by disease category as well as compounded annual growth rates, both projected for 2026, were discussed. Their findings were, in my opinion, confirmatory of my opinion about diet and health. The top categories in spending were:

- Oncology

- Immunology

- Diabetes

- Cardiovascular

- Respiratory

- Central Nervous System

But what was really revealing was the 5-year 2023-2027 CAGR spending (compounded annual growth rate) for each disease category. The results were:

- Oncology: 13-16 percent

- Immunology: 3-6 percent

- Diabetes: 3-6 percent

- Cardiovascular: 1-4 percent

- Respiratory: 3-6 percent

- CNS: 2-5 percent

Looking down the list, one finds the CAGR spending for two additional categories:

- Obesity: 35-38 percent

- Blood lipid regulators: 5-8 percent

These areas represent some of the highest CAGR for drug sales related to specific disease state categories in the coming years and should not surprise anyone. The CAGRs for cancer, obesity, diabetes, and blood lipids (cholesterol and other blood lipid elements) therapies rise as more people need these therapies (and admittedly are gaining access to the therapies). This is a result of many factors, of which diet is a primary driver. Certainly, there are other valid theories – environmental toxins being prime among them – that can explain the need for more therapies in these areas of disease, especially cancer and neurodegenerative diseases. But these trends are a mere extension of what I have observed in past research.

Please don't misunderstand. The drug companies have achieved great things, the rapid creation of anti-viral therapy Paxlovid for Covid-19 being perhaps the most recently dramatic. But let's not fool ourselves – the pharmaceutical industry may extend and improve lives *but it truly exists to make money*, for themselves and their shareholders. They are all too happy to be there with the solution when our diets, addictions and health habits lead us down the path of illness.

Big Pharma capitalizes on an all-too-common attitude among patients in this country. I call it the *pill crutch*. The pill crutch mentality is the attitude that you can indulge in what you know is health risky behavior as long as there's a drug to handle it. I see it all the time – among friends, patients, and fellow doctors. It is particularly common in statin use when it comes to controlling blood lipid levels. Now, statins have clearly made a difference in people's lives, particularly when there is a genetic predisposition to high blood lipids or concurrent cardiovascular risk factors like poorly controlled hypertension, heart failure, heart attack and the like. You'd be hard pressed to find a doctor who wouldn't treat with a statin any patient who fits the established guidelines for statin therapy. That would be risking the patient's health and life as well as inviting a malpractice lawsuit. What I'm talking about is a patient (or a physician caring for that patient) who will not try diet and exercise interventions before being prescribed a pill. I know that people think: "If the pill can take care of the problem, why can't I have the bacon cheeseburger with fries?"

And it's just this type of attitude – that a pill can handle what I throw at my body, even though I know what I am doing is unhealthy – that has contributed to the high number of medications we take and the potentially dangerous side-effects and interactions of those medications. Despite these side effects and "black box warnings" on some medications, people are seemingly willing to accept that as long as they can do what they want and act as they please.

Further evidence of Big Pharma's influence is the adjustment in treatment guidelines regarding certain disease states, particularly regarding the acceptable ranges of blood pressure and blood sugar. This is a controversial area, one I will not dwell upon here, but do realize that there is a large body of scientific literature that questions whether we physicians have unnecessarily lowered the acceptable ranges of blood pressure and hemoglobin A1C not because of scientific evidence but due to the influence of the drug companies. Critics have pointed out that the drug companies themselves are often the sponsors of such studies and therefore present a conflict of interest. For when the guidelines become tighter a new set of hypertensive and prediabetic patients are now created for the drug companies to market to and hook to therapy, much of it lifelong. How so?

Writing in the *Journal of Bioethical Inquiry* in September 2021, Linda Hunt, Elisabeth Arnold, Hannah Bell, and Heather Howard had this to say:

"Using diabetes as our example, we review successive changes over 40 years in screening, diagnosis, and treatment guidelines for type 2 diabetes and prediabetes, which have dramatically expanded the population prescribed diabetes drugs, generating a billion-dollar market. We argue these guideline recommendations have emerged under pervasive industry influence and persisted, despite weak evidence for their health benefits and indications of adverse effects associated with many of the drugs they recommend ..."

They go on to discuss the "pharmaceutical industry conflicts of interest" and "urge the development of a broader focus ... to curtail the systemic nature of industry's influence over medical knowledge and practice."

But whether the pharmaceutical industry's influence over research is overreaching or not, one thing is for certain – our reliance on prescription medication appears insatiable. A few statistics are relevant here. A study a few years ago by researchers at Mayo Clinic and Olmstead Medical Center found that 70 percent of Americans take at least one prescription medication and 20 percent of us take *five* or more. It is not that unusual for some Americans to take up to a dozen prescription medications, with the elderly dominating in this category. I once more quote former editor in chief of *The New England Journal of Medicine* Marcia Angell, as I have done in prior writings, from her 2004 book *The Truth About the Drug Companies: How They Deceive Us and What to Do About It*:

"... We have become an overmedicated society. Doctors have been taught all too well by the pharmaceutical industry ... to reach for the prescription pad. Add to that fact doctors are under great time pressure because of the demands of managed care, and they reach for that pad very quickly. Patients have been well taught by the pharmaceutical industry . . . If they don't leave the doctor's office with a prescription, the doctor is not doing a good job. The result is that too many people end up taking drugs when there may be better ways to deal with their problems."

So well said, particularly since the time that was written some twenty years ago, managed care has only increased in this country and people have gotten more unhealthy, not less. Sure enough, *U. S. Pharmacist* reports in the October 25, 2023 article "Americans Take Prescriptions a Large Portion of Their Lives" that about 85 percent of Americans 60 and older report taking at least one prescription medication in the prior month. They also quote an article that came out in the journal *Demography*, where Penn State researcher Jessica Y. Ho, PhD explained:

"There's a large body of research that shows Americans are less healthy and live shorter lives than our counterparts in other high-income countries. The prescription drug piece is part and parcel of that reality . . . the rates of prescription drug use in the United States are extraordinarily high."

The medications we take most bear a stark reflection of the state of our collective health. They are used, quite predictably, to treat the ailments that we suffer the most: cardiovascular disease, hypertension, diabetes, autoimmune disease, neuropathic pain, depression, and now obesity. Up until the rise of the new weight loss medications (see below) the most often prescribed medications in the past decade, according to a 2019 survey by GoodRX were:

1. Atorvastatin (Lipitor)
2. Levothyroxine (Synthroid)
3. Lisinopril (Prinivil, Zestril)
4. Gabapentin (Neurontin)
5. Amlodipine (Norvasc)
6. Hydrocodone/acetaminophen (Vicodin, Norco)
7. Amoxicillin (Amoxil)
8. Omeprazole (Prilosec)
9. Metformin (Glucophage)
10. Losartan (Cozaar)

Numbers 1, 3 ,5, and 10 deal with blood lipid/cholesterol control and blood pressure reduction. Numbers 4 and 6 cover acute and chronic pain, and number 9 helps with diabetes. I suspect the lineup has changed in recent years to reflect the rise of the new anti-obesity medications.

There's no doubt that the amount of processed and unprocessed food we eat here in the United States, combined with our increasingly sedentary lifestyles (see *Forbes*, a 2019 article by Nicole Fisher entitled "Americans Sit More Than Any Time in History and It's Killing Us"), are driving forces behind what Dr. Ho describes. Certainly, other factors are at play, but I think the evidence is clear. And much of the literature about Covid-19 infection has proven this to be the case.

During the pandemic, *The Economist* reported on June 24, 2020 some interesting findings that support my views.

"In hard-hit rich countries, about 60% of all deaths from the disease are among people 80 and older. America is an exception. Data released on June 16th by the CDC show's that the country's death toll skews significantly younger. There, people in their 80s account for less than half of all Covid-19 deaths; people in their 40s, 50s , and 60s account for a significantly larger share of those who die . . . Why is America such an outlier?...Americans may be less healthy than their European Peers, e.g., because they tend to be more obese."

More recent data presented in a *The New York Times* article of February 1, 2022 entitled "U.S. Has Far Higher Covid Death Rate Than Other Wealthy Countries" by Benjamin Mueller and Eleanor Lutz, proves how much less fit and resilient Americans are to weather the storms of the pandemic than citizens of other countries. They showed a graphic depicting cumulative deaths during the pandemic, in which The United States beat out Belgium, Britain, France, Sweden, The Netherlands, Canada, Japan, and Australia for the most Covid related deaths from January 22, 2020 to January 31, 2022. We were in the top spot again for cumulative deaths during the Omicron wave as well.

The authors quote a lagging rate of vaccination, as well as boosters, relative to the other nations. But it is this sentence that I feel is most revealing: "Many Americans have health problems like obesity and diabetes that increase the risk of severe Covid."

They present a graphic of how the Unites States leads in the obesity category over all the other mentioned nations.

You are free to draw your own conclusions. But the evidence is clear: The United States leads the developed world in the overweight/obesity problem. A heavily medicated society, people living in the U.S. are generally less able to withstand the rigors of a pandemic, we lag in many other health outcome parameters despite spending more than many of the developed nations of the world, and the numbers are getting worse with each passing year.

Instead of doing the hard work, instead of breaking the addiction cycle of processed food, UPF, higher body mass index and more sedentary behavior, instead of improving our lifestyles through concerted effort, we once again are relying on pharmaceuticals. This does not apply to everyone, for there are so many people who have earnestly tried everything within their power to control weight and are unable to do so. But for the rest who pin their hopes on these newer agents, real blockbusters designed not to treat the root cause of what ails us but instead to cover – like a bandage on a sore – the problem at hand, I say tread carefully. The following section speaks to just that.

What has been the typical American response to the crisis of high BMI? More drugs, of course.

Thirty-five years ago, the pharmacologic treatment of obesity was quite different. Back then the pharmacological buzz in the weight loss area was "Fen-Phen," the common name used for the combination of appetite suppressants fenfluramine and phentermine. The story of these drugs used in combination is a long and, in my opinion, sordid one. Yes, when used together these drugs did help people lose weight. In 1996 the FDA approved dexfenfluramine, a variant of fenfluramine. But all of a sudden, in July of 1997, reports came from the Mayo Clinic of patients developing serious heart valve problems and a rise in pulmonary (lung) blood pressure. Fenfluramine was taken off the market in 1997 and legal awards of billions of dollars were made to people (and their lawyers) who suffered ill effects from the drug. Since then, the drugs have virtually disappeared as an approach to drug-assisted weight loss.

Now, well into the twenty-first century, a new trend in pharmacologically assisted weight loss has swept the developed world and is especially strong in the United States.

Enter Ozempic, Weygovy, and Mounjaro, the money-making knights-in-shining-armor of the ever-increasing obesity epidemic. These drugs, and the other bioidenticals like Zepbound, are making headlines worldwide due to their ability to bring off weight rapidly. Tabloids and mainstream news outlets alike are full of stories of this or that celebrity who has dropped dozens of pounds and clothing sizes due to the actions of these drugs. People seemingly can't get enough of them (literally) and that is causing a relative shortage for people who really need them, the type 2 diabetics. People are paying 1000 dollars and more per month for the therapy, and I'm not only talking about customers who need to lose a lot of weight. There are reports of people who desire to lose 10, 15, or 20 pounds using the drugs, and plenty of doctors who are keen on the money-making potential of the off-label use of some of these agents.

Initially these drugs were developed to treat patients with type 2 diabetes and some concurrent conditions (also known as co-morbidities) such as chronic kidney disease and heart failure. Their utility was found to be related to their ability to either activate or block a receptor in the body relevant to blood sugar regulation and other parameters.

Jardiance (generic name empagliflozin) is an SGLT-2 inhibitor, i.e. it inhibits the action of a chemical in the body known as sodium glucose co-transporter-2. It is taken orally and treats type 2 diabetes as well as a form of chronic kidney disease and had been shown to decrease the risk of early cardiovascular death in some patient populations. It is not recommended in patients with type 1 diabetes and severe kidney disease. It works by blocking the reabsorption of glucose by the kidney tubules, thereby lowering blood sugar. It also fosters favorable heart muscle metabolism in patients with heart failure. Although not approved for this specific use, it can cause weight loss, although modestly so. There are serious potential side effects associated with its use, such as bladder pain, vaginal discharge, dizziness, low back pain, low blood pressure, abnormal blood lipids, fainting, painful intercourse, and most ominously a buildup of acid in the blood called ketoacidosis.

There are other drugs that do cause significant weight loss that also treat type 2 diabetes, and they are the focus of this section of the book. Monjauro (tirzepatide) is an injectable agent originally used to treat type 2 diabetes. Zepbound is the name of the weight loss version of the same drug and it has been used for weight loss purposes alone, where some patients have lost 21 percent of their body weight after 72 weeks of treatment. These drugs act as GLP and GLP-1 receptor (glucagon-like-peptide-1 and glucose-dependent insulinotropic polypeptide) agonists, meaning they *activate* certain receptor molecules in the body to achieve a desired effect. Those effects are known to:

- help the pancreas make more insulin
- decrease the amount of glucose (sugar) produced by the liver
- retard food passage through the gastrointestinal tract, making you feel full longer

It appears that the weight loss effect is dose dependent, that is, the higher the dose, the more weight lost. There are serious side effects that can occur, including nausea, diarrhea, vomiting, constipation, stomach and abdominal pain, low back pain, pancreatitis, and severe allergic (anaphylactic) reactions. People who have a family history of medullary thyroid cancer or a history of MEN-2 syndrome (multiple endocrine neoplasia syndrome type 2).

Ozempic (semaglutide) is a once-a-week injectable that mimics GLP-1, the naturally occurring hormone that causes insulin secretion from the pancreas and decreased glucagon production in the body. It was originally designed for treatment of type 2 diabetes and to decrease the risk of certain cardiovascular complications, but the form of this same medicine under the brand name Wegovy is approved for weight loss. Wegovy merely has more active ingredient than Ozempic, which is approved for type 2 diabetes management and not strictly for weight loss. Side effects can include low blood sugar, nausea, vomiting, diarrhea, dizziness, low energy, headache, sore throat, anaphylaxis, thyroid swelling, pancreatitis, and constipation. It carries the same thyroid cancer and MEN 2 warnings as Monjauro and Zepbound. There are even reports of stomach paralysis, as evidenced by an October 5, 2023 communique from the Faculty of Medicine at the University of British Columbia entitled "Weight-loss drugs linked to stomach paralysis, other serious gastrointestinal conditions." The communique based the headline on relevant scientific inquiry, saying "That's according to new research from the University of British Columbia showing that medications known as GLP-1 agonists – which includes brands like Wegovy, Ozempic, Rybelsus and Saxenda – are associated with an increased risk of serious medical conditions including stomach paralysis, pancreatitis and bowel obstruction."

It is not indicated for the treatment of type 1 diabetes.

Some of these agents have become extremely popular on social media and patients are increasingly asking for them. Many bariatric (weight loss) physicians are saying that in the extremely obese these therapies have been a boon for patients who have been unable to lose weight by diet and lifestyle changes alone. I applaud that. And there have been recent studies that support semaglutide's use in specific *subsets* of patients. For example, a compelling study in *The New England Journal of Medicine*, one of the world's premiere medical journals, appeared in the December 14, 2023 issue entitled "Semaglutide and Cardiovascular Outcomes in Obesity without Diabetes". There, authors Lincoff, Brown-Frandsen, Colhoun, Deanfield, *et al.* published their findings, which were achieved using the gold-standard double-blinded, randomized, placebo-controlled testing method. Double-blinded meant that neither the test subject patients nor the investigators knew whether the patients would receive the active drug (in this case, semaglutide) or a placebo, meaning an inactive solution potentially posing as medicine. The results were impressive:

> "In patients with preexisting cardiovascular disease and overweight but without diabetes, weekly subcutaneous semaglutide at a dose of 2.4 mg was superior to placebo in reducing the incidence of death from cardiovascular causes, nonfatal myocardial infarction, or nonfatal stroke at a mean follow-up of 39.8 months."

What was interesting about the study was that the patients were 45 years or older, had a BMI of 27 or greater and had no history of diabetes. The takeaway message was clear: the drug significantly reduced the incidence of death during the testing period from heart attack, stroke, and other cardiovascular disease. Bear in mind that the makers of the drug, Novo-Nordisk, sponsored the study. Also note that "more patients discontinued semaglutide than placebo because of adverse events, a result driven largely by a higher incidence of gastrointestinal symptoms with semaglutide" and that there was a major limitation in the study: "The diversity of the trial population did not duplicate a globally representative population; specifically, women and patients identifying as Black were underrepresented."

So, at least in patients with pre-existing cardiovascular disease, semaglutide appears to have utility in a restricted patient population. And the hidden inference in the results confirms in my view what I and many others have long believed and discussed; that both the Western diet-related and excess in weight in and of itself, independent of diabetes, worsens existing cardiovascular health, and most certainly aids in its creation in previously healthy individuals.

I have held these views in part due to the teachings of my late endocrinologist father Max G. Sherer M.D. and his mentor, one of the giants of twentieth century internal medicine, Isidore Snapper M.D.. Snapper was an interesting character. He was a Dutch physician, professor of medicine in China at the Peking Union Medical College around the time of the outbreak of World War II and was eventually taken prisoner by the Japanese, who exchanged his freedom for that of some Japanese prisoners who were regarded as highly valued. (Just before his release from the Japanese prison camp, he purportedly told the commandant of the camp, a man he allegedly despised, "You know, I am a famous doctor they are trading your soldiers for and let me tell you, you don't look so good.") He eventually came to Mount Sinai Hospital in New York City to teach where my father did his internal medicine training. Afterward training under Snapper in internal medicine my father ventured to The National Institutes of Health to complete a fellowship in endocrinology (that medical specialty that deals with glands, hormones and endocrine secretions from the thyroid, adrenals, hypothalamus, pituitary, and related glands). My father, like many physicians who knew Snapper, afforded godlike status to the man, and hung on his every word and teaching point. When questioned why he did not attempt to gain board certification in internal medicine by The American Board of Internal Medicine, Snapper famously quipped "Who would dare examine me?"

But in the vein of "whatever is old is new again" and "there is nothing new under the sun," the findings elucidated by the authors of *The New England Journal of Medicine* article on cardiovascular risk reduction and weight loss were reminiscent to me of what Snapper had surmised almost a century before in China. Snapper noted in one of his correspondences:

> "In 1940 . . . I confirmed the observation that in North China, coronary disease, cholesterol gallstones, and thrombosis (blockages caused by blood clots) were practically nonexistent among the poorer classes. They lived on a cereal-vegetable diet consisting of baked bread from yellow corn, millet, soybean flour and vegetables sautéed in peanut and sesame oil. Since cholesterol is only present in animal food, their serum cholesterol was often in the range of 100 mg. per cent. These findings paralleled the observation of De Langen that coronary artery disease was frequent among Chinese who had emigrated to the Dutch East Indies and followed the high fat diet of the European colonists."

Snapper later concluded that it was the diet high in vegetable oil, and not animal fats like meat, butter, and cheese, that afforded cardiovascular protection for the Chinese who stuck to their native diets and resulted in the higher unsaturated fats in their bloodstreams, particularly linoleic and linolenic acids. Snapper was also one of the first scientists to understand the importance of omega-3 and omega-6 in cardiovascular health. The man was decades before his time in thinking. His thoughts on plant-based diets and physical activity as a prevention of obesity and cardiovascular disease development were groundbreaking. They should be taught today in every medical school and shouted from the stages, rafters, and rooftops at every medical and public health conference.

Alas we live in different times, whereby the knowledge of giants is buried in the past and whatever the media can create a story behind is deemed sacrosanct.

Mindful both of Snapper's work and the exigences of the present times, I can see a use for these weight loss medications only in the direst cases of obesity and obesity with concomitant cardiovascular disease. For the rest of the populace who clamor to get their hands on these medications I have my doubts. It is exactly the wrong approach and wrong message to send to people who want to lose 10-20 pounds or even more weight quickly. The message instead should be to heed Snapper's observational wisdom; examine what you eat, look at your lifestyle and priorities and consider making some small and gradual changes.

Kate, the person depicted earlier this book, is likely to hear of these new drugs for weight loss and ask her doctor about them, Ted not so much. It's likely that Kate may have an employer-furnished health plan that might cover some costs of her medication therapy, and Kate, as a professional younger woman, might be more in tune with recent trends in healthcare and the drugs' media presence, to be aware of the perceived positives that people talk about. Ted, a working-class man in a rural area, with less formal education than Kate and probably a lower awareness of discussions around trends in health, medical treatments and physical appearance, might not know much about these drugs. However, as a veteran, Ted might be eligible under the Veterans Administration healthcare system, to receive Ozempic as a covered medication. Rest assured, the drug companies know full well who the potential users are out there and that there is money to be made, and lots of it.

The side effect profiles would be enough, one would think, that would discourage the casual use of these medications. There are risks to any medical therapy. But the wrong attitude has become all too pervasive: Why should I do the hard work when a medication can handle it for me? That's not me judging anyone, that's me speaking as a physician who has examined the scientific evidence, watched and listened to hundreds of thousands of patients in my forty years in medicine patients, knows that quick fixes often do not work, and that physiology was meant to operate in a certain way, honed over millions of years of evolution. I don't know about you, but treating my body well – and avoiding potentially risky laboratory- created molecular mimickers and blockers with an unknown long-term safety profile – is a better way to go. The problem lies in that not many people want to go that route.

But as more people turn to these medications for help, we are seeing reports of the potential dangers that come with their use. *CNN Health* reported in July of 2023 how women have suffered long-lasting gastric paralysis from Ozempic and Wegovy. CNN reporter Brenda Goodman had this to say:

"Doctors say that more cases like these are coming to light as the popularity of the drugs soared. The US Food and Drug Administration said it has received reports of people on the drugs experiencing stomach paralysis that sometimes has not resolved by the time it's reported."

In January of 2024, CNN again did a story on emerging cases related to complications from some of these medicines. CNN reporter Katherine Dillinger spoke of cases of hair loss, aspiration of stomach contents during anesthesia, and suicidal thoughts in patients taking Ozempic, Monjauro and Wegovy. The FDA is looking into these reports to see if any regulatory action is warranted.

And physicians increasingly are presenting case reports of complications from these medications. In my own specialty journal, *Anesthesiology News*, a publication for which I write a regular column, doctors recently recounted a case report of ketoacidosis (severe acid levels in the blood) after gallbladder surgery in a patient using empagliflozin, and another report of a young male patient who underwent esophageal and stomach endoscopy treated with semaglutide who was found to have food contents in his stomach even though he was on a pre-procedure fast. That patient was anesthetized and aspirated the stomach contents into his lungs, a potentially deadly complication. It was only through the excellent anesthesia care he received that allowed him to suffer no further complications.

Also in *Anesthesiology News* and *Gastroenterology & Endoscopy News* an article appeared on January 3, 2024, by Joe Morreale entitled "New Study Links GLP-1 to Severe GI AEs" (adverse events). In that report a previous study from the University of

British Columbia that had appeared in the *Journal of the American Medical Association* from October of 2023 was examined. In that retrospective study, which looked at the database records of 16 million patients from 2006-2020 who took either semaglutide or liraglutide (a related GLP-1 agonist medicine) versus an alternative treatment of naltrexone-bupropion for weight loss. The results revealed that those taking the GLP-1 medications had "increased risk for pancreatitis ... and bowel obstruction compared with naltrexone-bupropion ... The incidence of gastroparesis ... was also higher for the GLP-1 agonists" and "(T)he incidence of bowel obstruction was higher in patients on liraglutide." Gastroparesis means stomach paralysis or other contractile dysfunction. Commenting on these study findings, Eduardo Grunvald M.D., the director of the weight management program at the University of California, San Diego, said the agents "have potential serious side effects, and prescribers should be aware of them and feel comfortable managing adverse events, and understanding appropriate dosing strategies."

The previously mentioned University of British Columbia report from October 5, 2023 entitled "Weight-loss drugs linked to stomach paralysis, other serious gastrointestinal conditions" had also found these important relative risks when comparing the use of GLP–1 agonists to bupropion-naltrexone therapy for weight loss:

- "9.09 times higher risk of pancreatitis, or inflammation of the pancreas ..."

- "4.22 times higher risk of bowel obstruction" (blockage)

- "3.67 times higher risk of gastroparesis, or stomach paralysis ..."

But the drugs retain their popularity because our society is accustomed to immediacy. Why would anyone in a society that cultivates instant gratification choose to take a long-haul approach to solving a health problem?

The drug companies know their market well. They've done their research and recorded and analyzed their focus groups. Their marketing strategies are precise and based on analysis of their products, the influence they can have over physicians, and the message they can get to their target audiences – the doctor *and* the consumer.

People who stop these medications after an initial weight loss period almost always regain weight. Then they must stay on them indefinitely or are back where they started instead of fixing the problem for good, in a way more conducive to long term health and wellness.

I say once more: We do not know the long-term implications of these therapies because they are relatively new. Not many people are talking about that when the dollar signs are flashing and quick results are holding their attention. Will these medications eventually be shown to present more risks than they are worth, as was the case with phentermine in the late 1990s? In my opinion, more work needs to be done before employing these agents for moderate weight loss becomes the first line of action.

Aside from the bad food makers and the drug companies, a third group has emerged as a winner in this debacle – the makers of dietary supplements, meal replacements and the creators of app and web-based weight loss programs. According to a study presented by *Custom Market Insights* from April of 2023 entitled "U.S. Weight Loss Market, 2023-2032", the growth in this area is expected to rise from 135.7 billion dollars in 2022 to 305.3 billion dollars in 2030, a CAGR of 9.7 percent. The major players in this sector, such as Herbalife International, Nutrisystem Inc., Weight Watchers International Inc., and others have reaped the benefits of our increasingly high BMI populace and will continue to do so. The companies that provide the "weight loss supplements, meal replacement programs, fitness equipment, weight loss programs, and surgical procedures like liposuction and gastric bypass surgery" will continue to benefit as people flock to interventions that will partially undo or mitigate the damage they have done to themselves. They also point out the major trends in this growing area, including:

- personalized nutrition plans
- digital health solutions, through the use of smartphones and other digital devices
- plant-based diets
- behavioral coaching

The report confirms what I say now and have been saying for years:

"The high prevalence of chronic diseases, such as diabetes, hypertension, and orthopedic diseases, among the overweight and obese population is driving the growth of the weight management market . . . The rise in sedentary lifestyles, resulting from increased time spent in front of televisions and computers, has led to a higher incidence of chronic diseases among overweight or obese children. The consumption of junk food, physical inactivity and the growth of the fast-food industry have contributed to an unhealthy and sedentary lifestyle . . ."

Amen.

There appears to be a cyclical nature to our problem of bad food, overweight/obesity, and the influence of processed food manufacturers and Big Pharma. Academics and then the lay press decry the rise of weight-related health problems in our country, and worldwide. Panels convene, guidelines are discussed and set, politicians weigh in (think former First Lady Michelle Obama's campaign against childhood obesity and Congressional hearings on the diabetes epidemic and obesity in America with Charman Bernie Sanders, the WHO meetings on the global weight problem) and everyone gets hot and bothered. The food industry and the drug industry use their lobbying powers and their PR people to handle the issue under the guise of concerned, compassionate, and constructive action. The public muddles along, continuing knowingly or unknowingly on their journey with processed food and poor health. The noise quiets, new fads come along – promising this or that solution to our insatiable appetites – and the problem worsens, only to reemerge at some future time. Then we are at a higher set point, with a sicker populace, less people to care for them, and devoting a larger portion of our gross domestic product to cover the growing cracks in the dam.

The corporations make more money and the people, like the Kates, Teds, and the rest of us, suffer. But before you label me as a spokesman for a failed social experiment consider this: A lot of people are making a lot of money, as was and is the case with the tobacco and to some extent the alcohol industries, off the backs of an impressionable and chemically dependent public. Just as nicotine hooked generations of smokers, the processed food and UPF makers and the advertisers have taken us to where we are now. The situation is not tenable. Unless we all wake up to what is staring us in the face, it will be too late.

We are destroying ourselves on the micro level, both in our bodies and in our minds. The serious medical implications of what we are eating, how we use or don't use our bodies, and how we approach ourselves as animals, are factors many of us never consider in our all too busy daily lives. We are so desperate chasing what we fear we lack, the well-known FOMO (fear of missing out) phenomenon, that our health and well-being often take a back seat. The lay public, and the overly taxed doctors and other healthcare workers who care for us, have in a large part lost sight of what really matters in this discussion. We are first and foremost biological creatures, whose bodies and minds have undergone tremendous change in the last fifty years. Our tissues have been exposed to things that did not even exist a hundred years ago, causing a profound change in our immune systems, gut microbiome, brain chemistry, and metabolism. We assault our bodies every day with what we eat, how long we sit, and how we think. Our diseases, like diabetes, hypertension, and rheumatoid arthritis, are not merely metabolic, cardiovascular, or joint diseases, but more accurately *inflammatory* ones, brought on not only by genetic predispositions but our behaviors as well. And I will show the science to back that up. I ask that you keep these ideas in mind as we move forward with our discussion.

# PART 3

## Complications and Consequences

"You are the author of your own complications, and you can be
the author of your own simplicity."

**Carlos Wallace, Author of** *Life is Not Complicated, You Are*

On covers of the February 2021 editions of *Cosmopolitan* magazine,
there appeared some provocative photographs. Two women of
obviously high body mass index appeared in workout gear above
the headline "This is HEALTHY: 11 women on why wellness
doesn't have to be one-size-fits-all." The clear and important message, I believe, is a cultural one: People are individuals of worth and
should not be judged by their appearance. I agree with that. No one
with sense and sensitivity would or should think otherwise.

I must differ, however, with the scientific veracity of that
statement. As I have said many times before when it comes to

medical research and clinical evidence, science trumps sentiment every time. Medical literature is replete with science-based evidence that proves that high body mass indices are associated with the development of several well recognized and prevalent diseases, the very ones that I mentioned at the beginning of this book. Most certainly, there are slender people with both high blood pressure and diabetes, just as there are plenty of overweight people who have no other discernable medical problems. But the body positivity movement, like many contemporary movements, has embraced the concept that any *perceived* criticism or denigration of any chosen group of individuals (pick one) is unacceptable and merely part of an historically unjust and immoral construct, usually labelled as the *white male patriarchy*. Patriarchy or no patriarchy, we are steering people on a dangerous course, one that ignores science and favors political and social sensitivities.

I shall expend neither time nor effort in debating the validity or faults of such a concept, but I will say is that when it comes to objective science, I will place my bets on the scientific method and the accumulation and analysis of peer-reviewed evidence rather than whatever politically correct buzzwords or ideas happen to be in vogue. Social justice, a noble endeavor, should never reduce science and observationally derived truths to actions that are patently absurd. Consider the "don't weigh me unless medically necessary" cards that patients are handing their doctors and other caretakers and the preference for the term "non-adherence" over "non-compliance" with regard patients not taking medications as directed by the healthcare professional. One might as well, as a doctor or nurse, forego taking a pulse reading, blood pressure, oxygen saturation measurement and respiratory rate under such logic.

We should get something clear from the outset. Overweight/

obesity does not "cause" high blood pressure, diabetes, or joint disease any more than a solitary severe sunburn "causes" skin cancer. But the truism proven time and again in the medical literature is that high BMI is *associated with*, or *places you at risk* for, the development of a host of diseases, conditions that are becoming more common in the human population with each passing year. And since the premise of this book rests on the concept that what we eat is making us sick, it is incumbent on me as a scientist and physician to present you with the relevant research-derived evidence to prove to how this is so. You are free to discount or believe anything you wish. But I am hopeful and confident, notwithstanding the sentiment expressed by that revered and distinguished medical journal *Cosmopolitan*, that many of my colleagues would prefer that you heed my warnings.

Realize that there are two parallel pathways here guiding you towards illness: the effect of processed food directly on your body and the concomitant overweight/obesity state that often accompanies the ingestion of such products. Both areas have been the subject of extensive research and have been proven time and again to be deleterious to health on several anatomic and physiological fronts. But before we explore the ways in which this is so, let us dispel some common misperceptions about what many consider the primary ways in which illness is expressed in human populations.

### *How inflamed are you?*

Unless you've been living off the grid these many years you know that doctors have long warned of the dangers of high cholesterol, high blood pressure, diets high in fat, too much sugar consumption, diabetes, and the like. What you probably don't know is that the damage to the very organs and organ systems affected by these conditions and factors is probably not occurring the way you think it is. You should know that aside from blocked arteries, achy joints and arthritis, and high blood sugar there is a common thread that runs through the diseases that so commonly afflict us, and that is *inflammation.*

With each passing year, the inflammatory basis of disease has received more attention than perhaps any other area of medicine. And with good reason. The December 5, 2019 paper "Chronic inflammation in the etiology of disease across the life span" from the journal *Nature Medicine* by David Furman, *et al.* clues us in as to why this is so. In that paper the authors cite the very same diseases I listed at the start of this book – "cardiovascular disease, cancer, diabetes, chronic kidney disease, nonalcoholic fatty liver disease and autoimmune and neurodegenerative disorders" – that arise in part by what is known as systemic chronic inflammation (SCI). These disease states can arise by different mechanisms, some of the most prominent of which are "physical inactivity, poor diet, environmental and industrial toxicants and psychological stress." These stressors, as I have discussed earlier, are intwined with the consumption of an addictive diet of bad food and the physical inactivity that has become commonplace in our country.

This concept is not new in my writing, for in my previously mentioned 2021 book I had this to say:

> "A few decades ago, researchers studied inflammatory markers, particularly C-reactive protein (CRP), and found that the presence of high levels of these chemicals in the blood can be a good predictor of the development of coronary artery disease, heart attacks, and strokes. Doctors have long known of the correlation of subtypes of cholesterol in the blood (particularly LDL, or "bad

cholesterol") with those conditions, but a series of studies elucidated in *The New England Journal of Medicine* brought out the importance of CRP and the role of inflammation in cardiovascular disease."

My intention in stressing the role of inflammation is that we must not lose sight of how much this factor plays in ever-worsening contemporary disease, and how dependent our vascular health is on a diet that is as non-inflammatory as possible, that is, a diet that is the very antithesis of what most of us eat today. To best illustrate the importance of this statement, let me educate you about your vascular system, the very organ system that, when afflicted by disease, is responsible for more illness and early death than any other organ system in our body. Consider these facts about the lining of your blood vessels (the vascular endothelium) from the excellent book *Vascular Biology in Clinical Practice* by Mark Houston M.D.:

- Largest endocrine organ
- Largest organ in the body (!)
- Over 14,000 square feet surface area
- 6 ½ tennis courts in surface area
- 5 times heart size in mass
- Weight is 2 kg (about 4.4 pounds)
- Metabolically active
- Continuous sheet of parallel, polyhedral cells
- Releases vasoactive substances that regulate endothelial function, vascular smooth muscle, and circulating blood cells

- Major function: Maintain appropriate vasomotor tone (i.e. the pressure of the vessels), especially in coronary arteries and systemic resistance arteries

Think about it: When we attack ourselves with bad food and bad habits, the very lining of our body's circulatory highway is assaulted, bearing the brunt of the damage our addictions inflict upon it. There is no wonder why so many of us end up sick and dependent upon medication, particularly cardiovascular disease.

To best understand the health impact of our bad food and the concomitant obesity it entails we need to look at each organ system and relevant disease state. The US Center for Disease Control, the entity responsible for informing US residents about best health practices, had this to say:

People who are overweight (BMI 25 or higher) or obese (BMI 30 or higher) compared to those with healthy weight are at increased risk for many serious diseases and health conditions. These include:

- All-causes of death
- High blood pressure
- High LDL cholesterol, low HDL cholesterol, or high levels of triglycerides
- Type 2 diabetes
- Coronary heart disease
- Stroke
- Gallbladder disease
- Osteoarthritis
- Sleep apnea and breathing problems

- Many types of cancer
- Low quality of life
- Depression, anxiety, and other mental disorders
- Body pain and difficulty with physical functioning

I was not too far off when I called obesity "the mother of all diseases."

Let's take a closer look at the conditions that plague us to better understand the effect that bad food and/or high BMI have on our bodies. These I call the *micro consequences* of UPF and overweight/obesity. In the following section I will discuss the *macro consequences*, which relate to the environmental impact of producing processed food, the economic impact, and an area not well known the general public, our own military challenges with overweight and obese servicemen and servicewomen recruits.

## The Micro Consequences
### *Cardiovascular Disease*

Cardiovascular disease continues to be a major source of illness and premature death worldwide. The global epidemic of overweight/obesity fueled in part by the ingestion of bad food, sedentary lifestyles, and psychological stress, are primary drivers of this. But what exactly is going on in our bodies when we talk about this and why is it so important?

The circulatory system, comprised of your heart and all your blood vessels, from the largest arteries and veins to the smaller arterioles and venules all the way down to your capillaries, is the body's highway system for the transport of blood. Oxygenated blood, carried in the vast majority of your arteries (there are a few anatomical exceptions) is delivered to all the organs and tissues of your body in order to ensure their proper functioning and survival. Without getting too technical, the oxygen in your bloodstream, both bound to hemoglobin and dissolved into the blood itself, is a vital element that is necessary for animal life on this planet. We use the oxygen in the air we breathe for our metabolic needs and give off carbon dioxide by breathing it out of our lungs. This exchange keeps our organs and tissues healthy and helps to ensure the perfect acid/base balance (pH) to let all our enzymes, hormones, neurotransmitters, and other body chemicals work in an optimal state of conditions. Any deviations from the flow of oxygen rich blood to all areas of our body can result in disease and the worsening of preexisting disease.

In the case of the "Western diet" that my father's teacher Dr. Snapper alluded to 85 years ago, the buildup of cholesterol plaques or blockages, particularly in the coronary arteries (arteries that feed the heart muscle itself), the peripheral blood vessels (where blockages cause peripheral vascular disease) and in the brain and central nervous system (the location of "strokes" or, as it is called in medicine "cerebral vascular accidents") is a phenomenon familiar to most anyone. And it has been proven beyond doubt that diets high in saturated fat and refined carbohydrates place you at risk for developing these types of cardiovascular ailments.

In our own population in the United States, studies derived from autopsies of deceased young Americans from both the Korean War and the Vietnam War revealed the presence of arterial blockages in the coronary arteries in a small but significant number of servicemen. Part of the explanation for that was the prevalence of smoking, but it was thought that the longstanding American diet rich in saturated fat from a "hamburger and fries with apple pie and a shake" culinary mindset was a major contributor. The development of cardiovascular disease is complex and multifactorial with genetics, lifestyle and diet all playing roles as contributors. But in addition to the traditional medical thinking regarding the link between cardiovascular disease and high overall cholesterol, the dangers of "bad" cholesterol LDL (low-density lipoprotein), the deficiency of good cholesterol (HDL, high-density lipoprotein), and the excess of triglyceride (another blood lipid), other mechanisms related to oxidative stress, inflammation and secondarily to high BMI have been heavily researched and verified.

There are many possible mechanisms by which bad food and other UPF affect cardiovascular health. In their September 2021 *Advances in Nutrtition* paper "Ultra-processed Foods and Cardiovascular Diseases: Potential Mechanisms of Action", Juul *et al.* cite "absorption kinetics, satiety, glycemic response, and the gut microbiota" as well as "altered serum lipid concentrations . . . , obesity, inflammation, oxidative stress, dysglycemia, insulin resistance, and hypertension" and "neo-formed contaminants produced during micro processing" as possible factors in the cardiovascular disease association.

All of this is just a scientific way of saying that the consumption of processed food has been linked to:

- metabolically dysfunctional reaction of the body to the ingested food

- altered sense of fullness (remember Dr. Aronne from the introduction in this book)

- exaggerated glucose and insulin response to ingested food

- alteration of the healthy gut bacterial flora which helps regulate many aspects of health and wellness

- abnormal blood lipid profiles (Dr. Snapper's groundbreaking contribution)

- obesity and the other problems that accompany it

- inflammation, both systemic and localized, as in the hypothalamus

- oxidative stress, due to a deficiency of beneficial antioxidants and excess of harmful reactive oxygen forms (species) in the cells and tissues

- dysglycemia, or abnormal blood sugar levels, particularly in response to ingested glucose

- insulin resistance, that is a resistance to the normal action of the hormone insulin in the tissues

- hypertension, or high blood pressure, and the many complications that can result from it, including stroke, kidney disease, blindness, and peripheral artery blockages

It is easy to appreciate how incredibly complex and overlapping many of these dysfunctional states can be. But what should be apparent is that many mechanisms are at play with regard to high BMI, the inflammatory effect of bad food and damage to the cardiovascular system.

To their credit, Novo Nordisk, the maker of many metabolic disease medications, has been at the forefront of a movement to bring respectful and sensitive discussion about weight and health to light. Their campaign "Bring obesity to the forefront" is a great start, I feel, in opening an honest and caring discussion between patients and healthcare providers about weight. Their related website, www.rethinkobesity.com, is full of valuable information about the cardiovascular and other implications that higher BMIs carry. With reference to cardiovascular disease and obesity, they speak of the increased risk of high blood pressure, heart attack and heart failure, as well as the systemic inflammatory implications of high BMI, which may lead to "vascular breakdown, and cause structural and functional myocardial (heart muscle damage)".

When trying to visualize the damage to your circulatory system please imagine it this way. A healthy vascular system should look like a smoothly paved road, with no bumps, divots, potholes, or gravel to cause friction or a rough, jostling ride. Your vehicle on this road is powered by a pump, your heart, which beats against a steady but easily manageable head of pressure – like a mild headwind – as you travel. Along comes a diet of bad food and a lifestyle of inactivity and psychological stress and perhaps some other vices, such as smoking, illicit drug use and overuse of alcohol. Over time, things on the road and in your car begin to change, and not for the better. Your habits are impeding your travel and causing headwinds to build. That rise (hypertension) is causing your heart to beat harder and faster to fight the resistance it is facing. The diet and inactivity you embrace is causing chips, bumps, and small potholes along the highway (like the microtears from inflammation in your vessels and cholesterol blockages building up in your arteries) that add strain to your journey along the route. As this continues and the mechanical stress becomes too much the car, your heart muscle screams "I can't keep up with this!" and begins to strain due to a lack of oxygen to the heart muscle. The heart may even say "No more! I quit!" (heart failure) and your blood vessel highway, now accumulating more gravel and debris, is becoming blocked (plaque and inflammation) and now can't supply enough oxygen to your tissues. Before you know it, you have a heart attack (dead heart muscle) and a body on fire, full of inflammation, oxidative stress, blockages, organ damage and perhaps even worse.

This is what you are doing to your body every time you eat that double cheeseburger special, store-bought cupcake or 24-ounce soda. *When you watch a football game and the advertisements implore you to buy the fast-food poison to addict you further, you line the pockets not only of the junk food companies but the drug companies as well – all at your own expense. The ads on the evening news hawk all the pills and injections from Big Pharma to clean up the mess!* Think of that! You are paying for a slow death and a life full of medications all the while enriching others! You may not feel the effects right away, but over time, they'll get you. This is why it is so crucially important for your cardiovascular health to do everything in your power to resist these health-wrecking behaviors.

But it does not have to be this way. Much of the damage is reversible if changes are made in time. We will discuss that in part IV of this book.

## Diabetes, Metabolic Syndrome, and Prediabetes

To say that diabetes is out of control in our country is an understatement. The growth of this scourge has been astronomical, and the numbers tell it all. Once a relatively rare disease on planet Earth, it now affects so many people worldwide that The World Health Organization has sounded the epidemic alarm. And with good reason.

According to the CDC, 29.7 million Americans, or 8.9 percent of the population, has *diagnosed* diabetes. The numbers are surely larger due to unknown cases. Native Americans, Alaskan Natives,

Blacks, and Hispanics are particularly afflicted, as are the poor, less formally educated and those not living in a metropolitan area.

The journal *Population Health Management* from a February 2017 article entitled "Diabetes 2030: Insights from Yesterday, Today and Future Trends" by Rowley, Bezold, *et al.* warns that "the prevalence of diabetes (type 2 and type 1 diabetes) will increase by 54% to more than 54.9 million Americans between 2015 and 2030."

There is considerable misunderstanding about diabetes because we are really referring to different but often overlapping disease entities: type 1, an autoimmune disorder with some genetic component) and type 2 diabetes (a disorder at the whim of genetics, dietary and health habits, and our social environment). There are even hybrid forms of that display nuance with regard to symptoms, signs, characteristics, progression, and treatment. My late sister had type 1; she developed it at age 7, required insulin from that age onward and suffered a terrible progression of complications until her death at age 27. My father had type 2; he did not realize he was diabetic until his late forties, was treated with oral pill medication until his pancreas could no longer supply the insulin he needed and then required injected insulin until he died at age 87.

I will not go into the intricacies of diabetes and its pathologies, but it is important for you to understand that it is not merely a disease of a deficiency or absence of insulin, the hormone that helps blood sugar enter cells so it can give your body energy to work and help your liver store sugar for later use. Being diabetic can also mean that the body is not sensitive to the insulin it already has, a condition known as insulin resistance. But whether from a lack or absence of insulin production by cells in the pancreas, or an abnormal sensitivity to existing insulin, diabetes has been on the rise *in part* due to the food we eat, our sedentary lifestyles and other complex factors. High BMI places you at risk for the development of type 2 diabetes, as does the inflammatory and systemic stress of a diet of bad food.

But aside from being merely a glandular or strictly endocrine disease, where the pancreas is the primary focus, diabetes is a *vascular* disease, due to the effects of chronically high blood sugar, tissue inflammation and other factors. As in hypertension, diabetes that is poorly controlled can lead to what we refer to in medicine as end-organ damage, whereby target organs that rely on a robust and nourishing blood supply, like the kidneys, the nerves, the eyes, the gastrointestinal tract, and the heart, become damaged over time.

Because her diabetes was "brittle", my late sister Lisa suffered nearly all the diabetic complications of severe disease that one can experience: kidney failure (requiring dialysis and a failed kidney transplant), blindness, incontinence and nerve pain, stomach paralysis, frequent infections, and other tortures. It was the experience of watching a formerly promising young life snuffed out in such a brutal way that has made me the proselytizing health zealot that I am now.

My father's path with the disease was quite different. Although an expert in the care of diabetic patients he was unable to save my sister but was expert in preserving himself. He was able to live a relatively normal existence up until about the last two years of his life, golfing four times a week and working into his early eighties. He was able to prevent the end-organ damage that many type 2 diabetics develop in later life because he knew his body and he knew how to wield insulin. He was able to sense, without the use of a portable intermittent blood sugar monitor or a continuous glucose monitor that so many patients wear today how relatively high or low his blood sugar was and treat himself accordingly. If his sugar was too high, as evidenced by thirst and frequent urination, he'd give himself insulin. If his blood sugar was too low – feeling shaky, unsteady on his feet and tending toward confusion – he'd eat a candy bar, which he always carried with him. Eventually this ability gave out; I was once called on my cell phone by a man who had found dad lying in a ditch by the side of the road, barely coherent and fading fast. The man had pulled over and was at least able to call my number on my dad's instruction so I could tell the good Samaritan to get the Snickers bar out of the glove compartment and give it to him. Unfortunately, dad became more and more a brittle diabetic until the end of his life at age 87. Unlike my sister, he was able to avoid the horrific end-organ damage she had so painfully endured.

*Metabolic syndrome* and *prediabetes*, also rising at alarming rates in our country, are conditions that can be thought of as diabetes' precursor. Once again, bad food and bad habits put you at risk for these conditions, as does genetic factors. Metabolic syndrome occurs as a cluster of signs, particularly three or more of the following:

- hypertension
- high blood glucose levels
- high blood fats called triglycerides
- deficient levels of "good" cholesterol, or HDL
- a large waist size

Prediabetes, a possible precursor to diabetes, is thought to be present in **1 in 3 American adults**, about 80 percent of whom don't even know they have it. People with this condition have abnormally high blood sugar but not yet to the level that qualifies as diabetes. There appears to be a strong component of insulin resistance in this condition, and without preventive intervention both children and adults are at a high risk of developing diabetes itself. If you want to give yourself your best shot at avoiding the transition from prediabetes to diabetes it is clear that weight loss and an avoidance of processed foods, along with a diet low in saturated fat, refined carbohydrates, and sugar – and daily exercise – is your best course of action.

The message should be clear by now regarding both cardio-vascular and diabetes and its precursors: much of what you do on a daily basis involving what you eat and how you use your body and mind can have a profound effect on your risk of suffering these conditions.

### Neurologic Disease

There has been much attention in the scientific community directed toward processed food and the potential for developing or worsening neurodegenerative diseases, like Alzheimer's disease, Parkinson's disease, and amyotrophic lateral sclerosis (ALS). We have already discussed the behavioral and dietary factors that place you at risk for stroke, peripheral vascular disease, and coronary artery disease, but ongoing research has shed light on these other forms of neurologic dysfunction as well. Scientists have made the connection between obesity and the body's heightened inflammatory state and correlations have been made to this and the diseases I mentioned above, including multiple sclerosis. This is an exceedingly complex area of scientific inquiry, involving certain subcategories of blood cells and "pro-inflammatory factors." There is also ample evidence to suggest that both alterations in the gut microbiome due to dietary indiscretions and lifestyle choices play important parts in preventing degenerative neurologic diseases and in some cases slowing the progression of these disorders. Support for this connection between ultra-processed food and neurologic disease came from an April 1, 2023 article from *Harvard Health Publishing* in association with the Harvard Medical School entitled "Eating ultra-processed food tied to cognitive decline" by Heidi Goodman, and reviewed by Anthony L. Komaroff, MD. In that article, which made reference to a prior study from *JAMA Neurology* ("Association Between Consumption of Ultra-processed Foods and Cognitive Decline" by Natalia Gomes Goncalves, Naomi Vidal Ferreira, et al) that appeared December 5, 2022, Goodman states that there was "found a link between eating lots of ultra-processed foods and cognitive decline." She says that after "eight years, scientists found that middle-aged people who ate the most junk food had a faster rate (up to 28 %) of cognitive decline, compared with people who ate the least junk food." The researchers whose original paper had appeared in *JAMA Neurology* concluded that "Our findings are in line with previous studies linking consumption of UPF and adverse health outcomes, such as the increased risk of overweight and obesity, metabolic syndrome, cancer, cardiovascular diseases, and all-cause mortality."

As well, eating processed foods can alter the natural composition and function of beneficial gastrointestinal tract bacteria, microorganisms that are essential for proper metabolic function and good health. Because of this alteration in beneficial bacteria in the gut, inflammatory chemicals are released in the bloodstream and into the tissues which can promote or worsen degenerative neurologic diseases. The rise in the prevalence of these degenerative diseases is in part a result, I and many others contend, of the ubiquity of processed food and the increase in body weight circling the globe.

A paper in *Frontiers of Cellular Neuroscience* from November of 2023 by Neto, Fernandes *et al.* entitled "The complex relationship between obesity and neurodegenerative disease: an updated review" highlighted the contribution of low-grade inflammation in obese subjects to a higher risk of neurogenerative diseases. They say that since about 30 percent of the world's population is considered obese, countries across the globe are seeing increasingly prevalent obesity-associated diseases related to high body mass index, including neurogenerative diseases. They refer to the following factors as possible causes in this:

- hypertrophic adipocytes (oversized fat cells)
- a resultant triggering of inflammation
- followed by leptin and insulin resistance (remember our old friend leptin)
- blood-brain barrier disruption (meaning inflammatory chemicals can now enter the brain)
- neuronal inflammation
- brain atrophy (shrinkage) and cognitive decline

Again, we are seeing the "parallel pathways" I referred to earlier in this book: the inflammatory effect overgrown fat cells themselves in overweight/obesity (and its repercussions on health and wellness) *and* the direct inflammatory effect of the processed food. Certainly there are other factors involved here, such as the body's immune response to chemicals it had previously never experienced in thousands of years of human evolution, a subject I will address later in this chapter. But nevertheless it is important to understand that processed food *and* obesity in and of itself may pose deleterious effects on the well-being of both the central and peripheral nervous systems by way of multiple pathways and mechanisms.

## Degenerative Joint Disease

Your joints – particularly the weight bearing joints of your lower extremities and your spinal column – were designed to withstand a lifetime of stress. It is not difficult to appreciate both physical stresses of excess weight and the inflammatory effects of processed food both promote the development of degenerative joint disease and worsens existing joint disease. The odds are very good that you know someone who has had a total joint replacement.

Degenerative joint disease (DJD), also known as osteoarthritis, is a progressive disease usually associated with normal aging; most everyone will develop some degree of DJD if you live long enough. It is not to be confused with the other less common form of degenerative arthritis, rheumatoid arthritis, which is an autoimmune disease and has a different pattern of joint destruction, clinical implications, and disease progression.

DJD can affect many joints of the body, but the ones most impacted by higher BMI are the weight-bearing joints, in particular the hips, knees, ankles and joints in the feet and toes. Certainly, many people develop DJD in their fingers, hands, elbows, and shoulders, but since these do not bear as much weight as the joints of the lower extremity, they are less prone to the stresses of gravity.

The rise of lower-extremity DJD in our population is evidenced by the sheer number of hip and knee replacements, a clear correlate of average American girth increases. Indeed, a 2023 report ("Projections and Epidemiology of Primary Hip and Knee Arthroplasty in Medicare Patients to 2040-2060") in the *Journal of Bone and Joint Surgery* by Shichman, Roof *et al.* postulated estimates for future joint replacement tallies based on an analysis of past surgical utilization patterns. They surmised that between 2000 and 2019, the approximate annual volume of total hip replacement increased on average by 177 percent and for knee replacement 156 Percent. Relying on those estimates the authors projected that for each 5-year period going forward after 2020 the growth rate will be 28.84 percent for hip replacements and 24.28 percent for knee replacements. They say that this will cause increases in health care utilization and surgeon demand, something that will pose a challenge to our already overburdened and understaffed health care system.

It is estimated by the American Academy of Orthopedic Surgeons that every pound of body weight places four to six pounds of pressure on every knee joint. The AAOS also points out that people who are obese are twenty times more likely to need a knee replacement than those individuals who are not obese. Because obesity carries with it many of the complications I have already discussed at length, the AAOS is quick to point out the challenges and potential complications that may occur when replacing lower extremity joints, including "wound healing, infections, blood clots, blood loss, and dislocation of the replacement joint, especially the hip." That is precisely why joint replacement cannot be undertaken lightly and it is crucially important that concurrent illnesses like high blood pressure, diabetes, sleep apnea, and so on, be brought to optimal control through collaborative risk stratification by other physicians before anesthesia and surgery is performed. Formerly called medical clearance, this risk stratification means that a patient must be seen by other caretakers to ensure that all concurrent medical conditions are acceptably controlled. Failure to do so is a major factor in malpractice cases when things do not go as planned.

As an aside the recent opioid epidemic, partially fueled by the increased demand for orthopedic surgery, has been driven by the overuse and even cavalier dispensing of opioid medications. As I said in my 2021 book that enough opioid pills were doled out to patients in 2017 to give every American 32 pills. And we wonder why so many people suffered during that terrible time in American medical practice.

DJD will continue to be a major cause of pain and disability going forward if we do not get a handle on America's weight problem.

### Digestive Disease and the Gut Microbiome

Getting a better picture of how high BMI and bad food contribute to poorer health is particularly true in your own digestive tract. In the journal *Gut and Liver*, an international journal related to gastro-enterology, the medical discipline related to the digestive tract and related organs, author Su Youn Nam informs us in a 2017 article "Obesity-Related Digestive Diseases and Their Pathophysiology":

> "Obesity-related digestive diseases include gastroesoph-ageal reflux disease, Barrett's esophagus, esophageal cancer, colon polyp and nonalcoholic fatty liver disease, hepatitis C-related disease, hepatocellular carcinoma (liver cancer), gallstone, cholangiocarcinoma, and pan-creatic cancer."

The author goes on to explain the multifactorial causation of these diseases, including anatomical and hormonal factors as well as the inflammatory cytokines we have mentioned before in relation to other disease development. There should be a clear pattern emerging here: inflammation, oxidative stress, and the physiologic implications of carrying extra weight are all intertwined in a toxic brew of illness and disability.

Barrett's esophagus is a precancerous condition of the esophagus whereby detrimental cellular changes occur in the lining of the esophagus. It can be related to chronic acid reflux which causes damage to the cells that line the exposed interior surface of the esophagus and can be treated in some cases if it is diagnosed in time. Cholangiocarcinoma is a type of cancer of the bile duct, and I'm sure you have heard of pancreatic cancer, a disease that can be rapidly fatal depending upon the location of the tumor within the pancreas itself. Famous victims have included Patrick Swayze and Alex Trebek.

Nonalcoholic fatty liver disease (NAFLD) is a condition that is growing worldwide. It involves fatty infiltration of the liver and is a leading cause of significant liver disease in children, as is a more advanced form, nonalcoholic steatohepatitis (NASH). There have been correlations between the incidence of NAFLD and the increasing use of high fructose corn syrup, a sweetener commonly used in processed food. NAFLD is sometimes a precursor to inflammation of the liver and more serious liver diseases, such as liver cancer, cirrhosis (liver scarring) and outright hepatic (liver) failure. It turns out that metabolic syndrome itself is a risk factor for NAFLD, as is type 2 diabetes.

Writer Ann Lennon wrote in *Medical News Today* in 2022 that NAFLD affects about 24 percent of adults in the United States and that the condition is particularly prevalent among Mexican

Americans who consume large amounts of fructose, and other Hispanic groups as well. She reported that the degree to which fructose was present in the diet of Mexican Americans directly correlated to the incidence of NAFLD.

From my viewpoint the use of high fructose corn syrup as a sweetener by the processed food industry is one of the most sinister and despicable actions these companies have taken for the simple reason that the impact of their actions is so clearly damaging to the health of unsuspecting consumers, particularly children.

Robert Lufkin, a physician and adjunct clinical professor of radiology at USC Keck School of Medicine, publicly presented a dramatic graphic recently related to the soft drinks industry's use of high fructose corn syrup (instead of sucrose) in 1984 and the steady rise of NAFLD since then. He proposes that is when NAFLD really took off as a recognized disease entity and says today NAFLD is the *most common liver disease in the world*, a claim supported by the scientific literature. The switch to high fructose corn syrup in 1984 can be confirmed in a November 7, 1984 article in *The New York Times* by reporter Lee A. Daniels entitled "Coke, Pepsi to Use More Corn Syrup." The article delves into the beneficial financial effect of the switch for the soft drink companies, noting that "... the decisions underscore the long-building preference of the soft-drink industry for high fructose corn syrup – which is less expensive than the traditional cane- or beet- based sweetener – as well as the shrinking market of the sugar industry." There was absolutely no mention of the possible health effects of the switch and, to be fair, it is not clear when the detrimental health effects (metabolic syndrome, NAFLD, diabetes, etc.) of the sweetener were first recognized. Despite the incriminating evidence, however, high fructose corn syrup is still used today not only in making soda but in many processed foods as well. I think that is downright immoral.

The overconsumption of UPF has implications for another important area of general health – the gut biome. Our intestinal tracts, through countless thousands of years of human evolution, have been colonized with many forms of beneficial bacterial species. These bacteria, which are counted in the trillions of numbers in our bodies, contribute to a host of health-guarding functions, including (according to Zhang, *et al.* writing in the April 2015 edition of the *International Journal of Molecular Science*, "Impact of Gut Bacteria on Human Health and Diseases"): ". . . supplying essential nutrients, synthesizing vitamin K, aiding in the digestion of cellulose, and promoting angiogenesis and nerve function."

The authors say that based on the science, dietary and lifestyle choices – the very ones we are discussing in this book – can cause a condition called dybiosis, which in turn "can cause many chronic diseases, such as inflammatory bowel disease, obesity, cancer and autism."

The evidence is strong that our habits create yet another milieu in which our health is jeopardized from both an inflammatory and toxic point of view, all because of what we eat and how we behave. The angiogenesis the authors speak of refers to the salutary creation of new blood work networks, and the synthesis of vitamin K is crucial to proper blood clotting. In the case of autism, we see a proposed mechanism whereby our central nervous systems are negatively affected. Writing in the journal *Nutrients* ("The Western Diet-Microbiome-Host Interaction and Its Role in Metabolic Disease") in 2018, investigators Marit Zinocker and

Inge Lindseth found a damning link between UPF and damage to the gut microbiome.

In the case of UPF, obesity and the risk colon cancer, disturbing evidence continues to accumulate. As I noted in my 2021 book *What Your Doctor Won't Tell You*:

> "Sadly in our own country meanwhile, researchers have found an alarming rise in colon and rectal cancers in Gen X and millennial-aged people in our country. The reasons for this appear to be many. First, diets low in fiber and high in fat appear to be behind the increase in these cancers. Second, the resultant obesity from high caloric intake and a sedentary lifestyle was also cited by the researchers as possible reasons for the increase. Third, environmental toxins may also be playing a part."

Writing in the December 21, 2023 issue of *The Washington Post*, journalists Joel Achenbach and Laurie McGinley noted the trend as well in their article "Colon cancer is rising in young Americans. It's not clear why." They did allude to the possible role of obesity, "highly processed, low-fiber foods and a lack of exercise," as well as the fact that "systemic factors could be at work, such as changes in the gut bacteria – the microbiome – according to medical experts."

From a review of the literature, I would have to respectfully disagree with part of their headline. I think it is very clear why this is occurring.

## Obstructive Sleep Apnea (OSA)

If I were a betting man, I'd wager that the chances are great you know someone who has sleep apnea, either diagnosed or not. After all, the odds would be with me. Almost 40 million Americans have OSA, up from about 25 million in 2014. Estimates worldwide are in the range of 935 million people. If left untreated sufferers risk developing high blood pressure, cardiovascular disease, and early death. There is a clear correlation behind overweight/obesity and the incidence of sleep apnea, but even slender people can have it. The basic pathophysiology of the disease involves partial or complete obstruction of the airway during sleep, resulting in an increase in the activity of the sympathetic nervous system, a drop in blood oxygen levels, and the possible development of high blood pressure and cardiovascular disease.

There have been numerous studies linking the consumption of UPF and poor sleep quality, and many researchers have linked the consumption of UPF to both direct worsening of OSA and indirect worsening (through obesity) of the condition. A study published in *JAMA Open Network* in 2022 from Spain (Carneiro-Barrera, *et al.* "Effect of Interdisciplinary Weight Loss Intervention on Obstructive Sleep Apnea Severity") found dramatic improvements when a study group of overweight/obese men were placed on a weight loss and lifestyle change regimen. The lifestyle changes included "nutritional behavior change, aerobic exercise, sleep hygiene, and alcohol and tobacco cessation combined with usual care." A relevant fact was that the study participants were counselled to eat more vegetables and fruits, and other foods constituting elements of the "Mediterranean diet" replete with seafood, olive oil, legumes, poultry, and herbs. They were instructed to avoid the consumption of processed food as well.

The results were dramatic: "At 8 weeks, 45 % of participants in the intervention group no longer required CPAP (continuous positive airway pressure) therapy; at 6 months, 62 % of participants in the intervention group no longer required CPAP therapy."

No surprise there! Weight loss, exercise, avoidance of UPF, and nixing alcohol and tobacco abuse all contributed to a vast improvement in health, a reduction of blood pressure and weight, and fostered a sense of improved well-being.

Essentially, this experiment was clear proof of what I have been advocating in this book thus far.

### Autoimmune Disease and the Gut Microbiome, Continued

There's been a great deal of research dedicated to the increasing prevalence of autoimmune disease and the effect of bad food and high body mass index on both the development and worsening of pre-existing autoimmune diseases. Autoimmune disease, in which the body's own immune system attacks tissues and organs and thus causes disease and dysfunction, should be familiar to most anyone from either personal experience or who follows health and medicine. Your body's exposure molecules in the food, soil, air, and water are at play here because compounds created in the laboratory and not found in nature may cause your immune system to react as if these agents were foreign invaders set out to do harm. Important to remember is that it is not only the agents themselves that drive disease but the body's reaction to them that result in what I like to call the "drive-by shooter" phenomenon. Immune responses to the invaders and subsequent inflammatory reactions occur and – like innocent bystanders in a violent encounter – tissues and cells that just happen to be in the way get damaged because of the body's natural immune response.

Two hundred years ago an apple was just an apple, a handful of cashews was a handful of nuts and a piece of beef was merely cow muscle, sinew, gristle, bone, and fat. But today it is likely that the same apple is covered with diphenylamine, a chemical antioxidant that helps prevent the skin from degrading, fresh nuts may be riddled with chemical antioxidants like tea polyphenol and propylene glycol, and the beef you so enjoy on the grill is likely sourced from an animal pumped full of antibiotics and hormones. The very cooking of beef at high temperature can be associated with the formation of carcinogenic byproducts like heterocyclic amines and polycyclic aromatic hydrocarbons.

It is not difficult to envision that your body would recognize, after thousands of years of exposure to non- or minimally-processed food, additives in UPF as foreign elements that need to be neutralized by our immune systems. A casual examination of a box of processed cereal or a package of processed bakery goods reveals abundant chemical names that many physicians would find difficult to recognize. How do you think your own immune system is going to react to the myriad lab-created chemicals used in food processing? We already know the answer to that.

The American Autoimmune Related Diseases Association recently published some revealing facts about these set of diseases. The numbers are impressive – and worrisome:

- There are about 100 autoimmune diseases
- 50 million Americans have one or more autoimmune diseases
- 75 percent of affected people are female

- These diseases tend to cluster in families
- Some of the more common include lupus, rheumatoid arthritis, type 1 diabetes, multiple sclerosis, Crohn's disease, Hashimoto's thyroiditis, Grave's disease, psoriasis, celiac, sarcoidosis and ulcerative colitis.

The chances are very good that you know someone with auto-immune disease, and that fact along with the growing number of people suffering from them has created a lot of buzz in the world of science and in popular media. A 2022 article in *The Guardian* and *The Observer* by Robin McKie entitled "Global spread of autoimmune disease blamed on western diet" looked at the work of two scientists from London's Francis Crick Institute, James Lee, and Carola Vinuesa. Invoking possible changes in the gut microbiome, Vinuesa believes that as more countries adopt a western diet heavy with fast food, the more autoimmune disease we are see. She said:

> "Fast-food diets lack certain important ingredients, such as fibre, and evidence suggests that this alteration affects a person's microbiome ... These changes in our microbiome are then triggering autoimmune diseases, of which more than 100 types have now been discovered."

She pointed to genetic predispositions to the development of autoimmune disease that may become "unmasked" when the microbiome is negatively affected by a western-style diet. Chris Van Tulleken concurs in his book *Ultra -Processed PEOPLE, The Science Behind Food That Isn't Food*, citing a form of "leaky gut" whereby the altered microbiome (dybiosis) of the intestines leads to damage to the important gut barrier. This barrier is formed by "tight links between cells, mucus and immune cells." The result is that "the gut starts to leak microbes and their waste products into the rest of the body." He refers to two possible food emulsifiers – carboxymethyl-cellulose and polysorbate 80 – as possible culprits in dybiosis.

Again we see the themes of inflammation, an altered microbi-ome and processed food as likely suspects in the creation of human disease.

## Cancer

The *World Cancer Research Fund International* calls the growing global burden of cancer one of the "most significant public health challenges of the 21st century." With the increase in bad food con-sumption, more sedentary lifestyles, increasing body weight, and the continued abuse of tobacco and alcohol, this should surprise no one. The organization revealed that in 2020, 18.1 million cases of cancer were reported worldwide, with 9.3 million cases in men and 8.8 million cases in women. The most prevalent types of cancer were breast and lung cancer, followed by colorectal, prostate, stom-ach, liver, cervical, esophageal, and thyroid cancer.

There are untold number of studies linking diets rich in saturated fat and refined carbohydrates to many forms of cancer, and now there is compelling evidence that a diet high in UPF is a main contributor as well. Writing in the British medical journal *The Lancet*, Chang, Gunter, Rauber et. al. found in their January 2023 article "Ultra-processed food consumption, cancer risk and cancer mortality: a large-scale prospective analysis within the UK Biobank":

"First, every 10 % increment in UPF content of diet was associated with an increased incidence of overall cancer by 2% and ovarian cancer by 19%. Second, participants with the highest compared with the lowest UPF consumption quartile had a higher incidence of overall and brain cancer, and a lower incidence of head and neck cancer. Finally, every 10% increment in UPF consumption was associated with increased mortality of overall cancer by 6%, breast cancer by 16%, and ovarian cancer by 30%. These associations persisted after adjustment for a range of key socio-economic, behavioral and dietary factors."

The keys factors to realize in this valuable study are that:

- the more the diet consisted of UPF, the higher the incidence of cancer itself.

- the more the diet consisted of UPF, the worse was the death rate from any particular form of cancer.

- even adjusted for lifestyle, economic and social status, and other dietary factors, the positive correlation of UPF to cancer remained.

Of interest is what the authors say later in the article:

". . . dietary patterns with a high UPF content are generally nutritionally inferior and are higher in energy, total and saturated fats, salt and free sugars, and lower in fibre and several micronutrients . . . furthermore, evidence has been accumulating on the strong obesity and type 2 diabetes – promoting potential of UPFs, both of which are risk factors for many cancers including those of the digestive tract and some hormone-related cancers in women."

The authors also mentioned the more well-known links to cancer and diet, including artificial sweeteners, nitrates and nitrites, acrylamide formation during high temperature cooking, and phthalates and bisphenols (remember those?) from food storage, packaging and contacting materials.

As I said earlier in this book, artificial things abound in the world we live in and when it comes to ingesting chemicals that did not exist 200 years ago the body very likely sees the new molecules as invaders that need to be dealt with. It seems that changes to the microbiome and bystander-type tissue damage from inflammation and oxidative stress correlate with both the development of cancer and the worsening of existing cancer diagnoses.

## Psychiatric Disease

The link between UPF and psychiatric disorders has been widely studied in the medical literature and there is growing evidence that disorders as diverse as depression, anxiety, attention deficit disorder, autism, and even schizophrenia may have some connection to the food we eat. For example, a September 2023 article in *The Guardian* by Ann Bawden entitled "Ultra-processed food linked to higher risk of depression, research finds" summarized a large American study on this topic. Researchers at Harvard Medical School and The Massachusetts General Hospital examined the diets and mental health of 30,000 women over a 14-year span. Their conclusion was:

"Adjusting for other health, lifestyle and socioeconomic risk factors for depression, the research, published in the US journal JAMA Network Open, found that those who consumed nine portions or more of ultra-processed foods a day had a 49% increased risk of depression compared with those who consumed fewer than four portions a day."

They found that artificial sweeteners in soft drinks and other drinks were particularly significant in that these substances may "trigger the transmission of particular signaling moleclues in the brain that are important for mood."

Other investigators have found a similar link between UPF and depression. In the journal *BMC Medicine* from April of 2109, the article "Prospective association between ultra-processed food consumption and incident depressive symptoms in the French NutriNet-Sante cohort" by Adjibade *et al.* found a correlation between depression and sweeteners in drinks, sauces, and added fats in a study of almost 27,000 subjects aged 18-86 years. What was really interesting in the study was this information:

"In particular, a recent meta-analysis of including 21 studies conducted in 10 countries reported that a diet rich in red meat, processed meat, refined grains, sweets, high-fat dairy products, butter, potatoes, and high-fat gravy was associated with an elevated risk of depression ..."

The authors noted the possible role of "additives (in particular emulsifiers) or molecules resulting from high-temperature heating which may among others cause alterations in the gut microbiota which has been suggested to show important interrelations with mental health."

Since this was a prospective study, using a large sample size, "repeated assessment of depressive symptoms using a validated tool", and meticulous attention to the dietary data in the study, the investigators expressed confidence about the validity of their conclusions. The fact that they analyzed data from a "meta-analysis" adds strength to their findings since such a "study of studies," whereby much data and scientific evidence has been collated from multiple sources, tends to increase the value of the findings and the proposing of new hypotheses.

Other psychiatric conditions and their possible link to UPF have been examined as well. Attention deficit disorder, anxiety, and even autism have been linked to diets overabundant in UPF. Some of these disorders, it has been proposed, are being seen more frequently because of weight gain in children and the resultant proinflammatory effect of hypertrophic fat cells. Another mechanism proposes that certain preservatives in UPF may be partly to blame. Some investigators propose that mothers who eat a high UPF diet during pregnancy are potentially risking the mental health of their offspring, especially regarding the later development of autism.

A key point to understand is that there exists a gut-brain axis in every human being, whereby the intestinal bacteria interact with both the central and gut-related nervous systems. The common phrases "trust your gut" and "what's your gut feeling on this" portrays this all too well. From the journal *Annals of Gastroenterology* ("The gut-brain axis: interactions between enteric microbiota and enteric nervous systems") in April of 2015, scientists Marilia Carabotti et. al. described this essential interaction:

"The gut-brain axis (GBA) consists of bidirectional communication between the central nervous system, linking emotional and cognitive centers of the brain with peripheral intestinal functions. Recent advances in research have described the importance of gut microbiota in influencing these interactions."

Keeping that in mind, you can better appreciate the importance of the GBA in a psychiatric disease as prickly and devastating as schizophrenia, where some investigators have alluded to a disruption of this axis and effects on the microbiome as possible contributors to the development of this condition. In their paper "Schizophrenia and obesity: May the gut microbiota serve as a link for pathogenesis?" Hui Wu *et al.* said in an *iMeta*, Volume 2, issue 2, April 4, 2023 article "Schizophrenia and obesity: May the gut microbiota serve as a link for the pathogenesis?" that schizophrenic patients are more likely to develop obesity than non-schizophrenics, that maternal obesity during pregnancy is associated with a higher chance of having a schizophrenic offspring, and that gut dybiosis can cause "immune inflammation" which in turn is related, it is thought, to "the onset of schizophrenia and obesity through shared pathophysiological mechanisms . . ."

Most promising in this article was the line "Gut microbiota is a modifiable component that may be used as a novel therapeutic approach for treating obesity or improving outcomes in schizophrenic patients" This means that treatments that foster healthy intestinal bacterial populations in just the right amount might favorably influence outcomes in weight management and schizophrenia.

The thought that by positively impacting the gut microbiome we might be able to take a new therapeutic approach to both obesity and a serious debilitating psychiatric disease is extremely exciting.

## Fat and Muscle as Endocrine Organs

According to scientists Marisa Coelho, Teresa Oliveira and Ruben Fernandes, (*Archives of Medical Science*, April 2013 "Biochemistry of adipose tissue: an endocrine organ") fat, also known as adipose tissue, is not merely a repository of what many consider aesthetically displeasing but an organ itself that "exerts an impact on whole body metabolism" and is "responsible for the synthesis and secretion of several hormones" that are "active in a range of processes, such as control of nutritional intake (leptin, angiotensin) control of sensitivity to insulin and inflammatory process mediators . . . and pathways."

They go on to describe the difference between brown fat and white fat. Brown fat is relatively scarce in adult humans and is important for heat production (thermogenesis). The brown fat cells are generally smaller than white fat cells, and the latter's "capacity is much broader and more comprehensive" than brown fat. White fat:

- has a more extensive distribution in the body, even in the organs, abdominal cavity, and muscles

- acts as insulation

- can "accumulate and provide energy when necessary: and is "important for lipid energy balance, particularly fatty acids, which are an exceptionally efficient fuel source species."

- "is dynamically involved in cell function regulation through a complex network of

endocrine ... paracrine ... and autocrine signals
that influence the response of many tissues including
hypothalamus, pancreas, liver, skeletal muscle, kidneys,
endothelium and immune system ..."

The important point in their article is that "... unbalanced production of pro- and anti-inflammatory adipocytokines in obese adipose tissue may contribute to many aspects of metabolic syndrome ..."

In plain English, that means that an abundance of fat can produce chemical agents that may be responsible for inflammation and subsequent development or exacerbation of metabolic syndrome, a pathologic entity I described previously. Truly, a "battle of the bulge!"

Muscle tissue has now been considered by many as an endocrine organ itself, responsible not only for movement, postural support, and the performance of physical labor, but also as an "energy production and consumption system that influences the whole body's energy metabolism ... skeletal muscle synthesizes ... myokines" which "exert beneficial effects on peripheral and remote organs." (Kenzi Iizuka *et al., Journal. Pharmacol. Science,* May 23, 2014 ("Skeletal muscle is an endocrine organ"))

Restated, these chemicals called myokines exert influence in other parts of the body to maintain health and homeostasis.

You might ask why this is relevant to our discussion. The reason is that many studies have conclusively confirmed that the ingestion of diets high in UPF, as well as a sedentary lifestyle, encourage the accumulation of excess body fat. This changes the composition of the body's lean/fat ration and has implication in the development of human disease states. For example, we have already discussed the pro-inflammatory and microbiome-damaging effect of excess body fat. But the body gets a "double whammy" when the amount of ingested UPF reaches a certain threshold, simply because many studies have correlated a high UPF diet with loss of muscle mass itself. This causes physical deconditioning, resultant postural changes, and a diminution in the ability to perform physical labor. But most importantly the loss of muscle mass *per se* (also called sarcopenia) is associated with poor health outcomes in several ways. From the *Journal of Clinical Nutrition* in November of 2023 came this paper by Robinson, Granic, *et al.* entitled "The role of nutrition in prevention of sarcopenia." There the authors concluded that:

> "Diets of higher quality, characterized by the frequent consumption of fruits, vegetables, wholegrain foods, legumes, and fish, but *lower consumption of highly processed foods* (italics mine), are linked with a range of health outcomes ... associated with a lower risk of noncommunicable diseases including cardiovascular disease, diabetes, cancer, and all-cause mortality. The recent growth in dietary pattern studies indicates the potential beneficial effects of higher quality diets for muscle function in older age, particularly linked to better-measured physical performance in older age.

> "However, healthier diets of higher quality across adulthood, with known benefits for a number of health outcomes, are also linked to preservation of muscle mass and function – with the potential to enable better physical performance and independence in older age."

Many investigators ascribe to the existence of something known as sarcopenic obesity (SO), a condition in which obesity and a loss of muscle mass coexist in the same individual. This condition has been found to be particularly prevalent in the elderly and is a significant cause of chronic disease and disability. Some studies suggest that fat and muscle tissue also engage in cross talk, a way of bilateral communication through proteins (adipokines and myokines) secreted by both adipose and muscle cells themselves. Kristin Stanford and Laurie Goodyear discussed this in their August 2018 article "Muscle-Adipose Tissue Cross Talk" which appeared in *Cold Harbor Perspectives in Medicine.* In that article the authors quote studies that confirm that serum leptin levels correlate to the amount of fat tissue a person has. You will recall our discussion of leptin at the beginning of this book, and how it is chronically elevated yet dysfunctional in overweight/obese people who have hypothalamic inflammation from diets rich in saturated fat, refined carbohydrates, and sugars (which is known to be abundant in much fast food and UPF). The authors found that exercise training "results in profound changes in white adipose tissue, including an altered profile of both myokines and adipokines." They emphasize that "Given the increasing prevalence of obesity and type 2 diabetes, human exercise studies will be critical to gain further insight into the function of novel adipokines and define their role in skeletal muscle and whole-body metabolism . . . Exercise-induced adipokines may have additional benefits on overall health beyond glucose metabolism and could be interesting novel therapeutic targets for obesity, type 2 diabetes, and other diseases."

These studies confirm what common sense has long told us: less body fat (from eating a balanced, un- processed diet in moderation) and more muscle (achieved through exercise) are good for you.

## The Macro Consequences

### *The Environmental Impact*

The environmental impact related to the production of processed food is an exceedingly complicated and nuanced topic, one that has received a great deal of attention in recent years. You could easily spend an entire book on this topic and the research behind the theories drawing upon many disciplines, including environmental biology, animal science, sociology, psychology, economics, anthropology, and geology. The production of UPF has been called a threat to our planet's agrobiodiversity, a concept that relates to the environmentally beneficial and health-promoting effects of drawing our food sources from diverse, balanced, and sustainable sources. I have mentioned Chris Van Tulleken's book before and I refer you to his section on the topic for a deeper understanding of the issues. Some of the key points he makes in that part of his book are:

- "UPF is a particular driver of carbon emissions and environmental destruction."

- If diets tend to remain relatively the same, greenhouse gases will nearly double by the year 2050.

- "Just twelve plants and five animals now make up 75 % of all the food eaten and thrown away on the Earth."

- The dominant food on the planet presently is vegetable oil, especially palm oil, of which three-quarters is used in UPF production.

- "Since 1970, more than half of all the virgin rainforest in Indonesia has been destroyed for palm oil." This has resulted in astronomical levels of carbon emissions, such that ". . . the fires in 2015 emitted more carbon dioxide than the entire United States economy" on several distinct days.

- The current food global production system is enormously expensive because "according to the International Monetary Fund and lots of other people, we all subsidize it by paying around 6 trillion USD worth of external costs, like increases in healthcare costs due to air pollution and the costs of a changing climate."

- To hasten production times, animals are now fed higher nutritional-value plants, as opposed to feeding them "very low-quality plant protein" such as grass, leaves, food waste, and forage.

- Meat as a food source is much less carbon friendly (production wise) to the environment than plants.

- Chicken is the world's most popular meat source. The "birth-to-slaughter time for 95% of the chicken we eat is just six weeks . . . These chickens are fed on a high-protein diet of some fishmeal and a lot of soya . . . Each year, 3 million tons of soya are imported to the UK, and most of it has caused environmental destruction that is already affecting the global climate."

He goes on to say that because meat production will almost double by 2050, vast amounts of land will be required to produce the corn and soy to feed the livestock, an area "the size of Europe" itself. Indeed, Van Tulleken also makes a point of the pesticides used in feeding these sources of meat-based protein, and the resultant "birth defects and higher cancer rates among local populations." He alludes to the fact that since massive deforestation and clearing of the land is needed to farm the agricultural products to feed the animal sources of protein on a large scale, you get less rain because there are less trees to "'breathe out' water vapor, which creates new clouds that travel further inland . . ." This causes a vicious cycle of foliage destruction, increased industrial farming, reduced tree-based water vapor production, and drought. He closes his section by pointing out the effect of widespread antibiotic use in animal farming and its negative impact on human health through antibiotic resistance, as well as the impact of plastic exposure. He referenced, according to Break Free From Plastic's yearly audit, Coca-Cola, PepsiCo, and Nestle as 2020's global leaders in plastic pollution. And this in itself has grave consequences for human health.

The findings of other investigators support Tulleken's narrative. Fifty-two studies were examined in a recent paper in the July 2022 *Journal of Cleaner Production* article "A conceptual Framework for understanding the environmental impacts of ultra-processed foods and implications for sustainable food systems" (Anastasiou, Baker, *et al.*). They cited similar threats to the global environment, and their findings are summarized here:

> "UPFs accounted for between 17 and 39% of total diet-related energy use and 36-45% of total biodiversity loss, up to one-third of total diet related greenhouse gas emissions, land use and food waste and up to one-quarter of total diet-related water use among adults in high income countries . . . The findings highlight that environmental degradation associated with UPFs is of

significant concern due to the substantial resources used in the production and processing of such products, and because UPFs are superfluous to basic human needs."

The relevance of plastics and their effect on human health is equally chilling. Plastic is everywhere in our world, from the deepest depths of the oceans to the highest mountaintops. Ubiquitous in diverse societies around the globe, plastic is used to contain our drinks, package our food, in the construction of our consumer products, our toys and gadgets, and our babies' pacifiers. I mentioned earlier the three major plastic polluters according to a recent survey, but what exactly are the health implications for this seemingly universal entity?

From an April 18, 2022 report from *Henry Ford Health* comes this:

"About 77 % of the people who were tested were found to have microplastics in their bloodstream . . . Here are just a few issues that microplastics may be causing:

—Microplastics may act as endocrine disruptors . . . blocking the effect of our own hormones . . . it could lead to fertility issues, blood sugar imbalances, metabolic issues, hypothyroidism and hyperthyroidism, autoimmune diseases – and much more.

—Microplastics may contribute to cancer."

The respected medical oncologist and hematologist Philip Kuriakose of Henry Ford Health was quoted as saying, relative to the increased risk of cancer, that "Our bodies are very dependent on our ability to repair damages. Our cells are constantly regenerating and we're dying a thousand deaths every day, but we don't realize it because our genes are often able to suppress those abnormal, cancer-causing cells. But if microplastic are interfering with cell regeneration, it may cause a higher incidence of cancer and other diseases."

You may ask why this has special relevance for processed food. First, most fresh, organic, unprocessed food can be contained and/or transported in paper bags, or other non-plastic containers. Any purchase at a farm market or roadside stand is evidence of this. Even if the food is taken home in a plastic bag, the exposure time to the plastic itself would be limited. Second, we all are aware of the high amount of plastic used in packaging UPF. The magazine *Wired* presented a provocative article by Celia Ford in July of 2023 appropriately entitled "For the Love of God, Stop Microwaving Plastic." In that article she described how microwaving food in plastic "delivers a double whammy: heat and hydrolysis, a chemical reaction through which bonds are broken by water molecules. All of these can cause the container to crack and shed tiny bits of itself as microplastics, nanoplastics and leachates, toxic chemical components of the plastic."

The article in *Wired* reconfirmed some of the points made in the Henry Ford article about the potential for human disease causation and plastic exposure.

The bottom line is that plastic quite likely is causing a threat to human health and that, because of our exposures to plastic in UPF, we all need to be mindful of this additional health impact, especially with regard to microwaving processed food in their as-sold containers.

## The Economic Impact

Worldwide, the economic impact of UPF – and its frequent bed-fellow overweight/obesity – is as significant and devastating as their personal and environmental effects. This is particularly true in the United States, which spends more per capita on health care than any other nation. Statista.com reports that in 2021, the total amount spent to cover healthcare costs in our country was over 4 trillion USD and that as a percentage of gross domestic product, that figure will increase by 20 percent by 2031. The Commonwealth Fund reports that despite our highest level of spending per capita we place dead last with regard to measures of quality, efficiency, access, equity, and the promotion of longer, healthier lives among when compared to Australia, Canada, Germany, the Netherlands, New Zealand, and the United Kingdom. You might wonder why this is so.

That is a difficult question to answer, but socio-economic history can be illuminating. Long an industrial powerhouse, the United States has long been a leader in innovation, creativity, and mass production ever since the latter part of the nineteenth century, bringing the airplane, automobile, and telecommunications to much of the world. The robber barons of the late 1800s and early 1900s wielded their incredible wealth and leveraged their power to not only dominate world production of consumer goods and services (think Cornelius Vanderbilt, Jay Gould, Henry Ford, Andrew Carnegie, John D. Rockefeller, Leland Stanford, and the like) but to spread their influence beyond the lucrative businesses related to transportation, energy, and industrial materiel. Men like C. W. Post., W. K. and Dr. John Harvey Kellogg, Asa Griggs Candler, as cereal makers and soft drink manufacturers respectively, were to the food and drink and non-alcoholic beverage industry what Henry Ford and the Dodge brothers were to the automobile.

As America spread its food and beverage products across the country and then the world, our nation became the beacon of industrial mass-production and a shining example of successful capitalism. Even the dictator, despot, and mass-murderer Adolf Hitler expressed his extreme envy for the economic might and the unbridled innovative capitalistic drive of the United States before our country entered the war to defeat Naziism, Fascist Italy, and the Empire of Japan in 1941. Americans were rapidly becoming a nation that liked to do things in a big way and blessed with an incredibly diverse and large land mass in terms of natural resources and agricultural capabilities, the United States soon found itself leading the world in the production of processed food.

After the Second World War America settled down to a new era of prosperity. During the 1950s, we witnessed the expansion of the suburbs, the continued popularity of the automobile, and the rise of fast food along the inter- and intrastate highways. The rising prevalence of processed food in American supermarkets, along with the appearance of the TV dinner (to accompany the growth of television itself as a quintessential form of American entertainment) gave way to a new way of eating habits. Fast food giants like McDonald's, Burger King, Kentucky Fried Chicken, and countless others (along with the ubiquitous diners) dominated their sector of the food industry along the highways and in the small, medium, and large towns and the cities all over the United States.

At the same time, technological innovation began its meteoric rise. Companies like International Business Machines (IBM), Hewlitt Packard, General Electric, Westinghouse, and so many others laid the foundation for the future tech giants of the likes of Microsoft, Apple, Dell, and Oracle. This paved the way for a change in the very nature of labor itself. Gone were many jobs that required sheer physical labor; the back-to-back revolutions of the "computer age" and the "internet age" completely reshaped the way people in the U.S. worked, and as a consequence, the way Americans moved their bodies.

Today, much like it was in the twentieth century, the United States is a nation of commuters, and walking as a means of daily transportation has taken a back seat to the car, bus, subway, and train. But unlike before, more people are staying home to do their jobs than ever, particularly in light of the Covid-19 pandemic. According to a census.gov report from September 2022, statistician Michael Burrows said, "With the number of people who primarily work from home tripling over just a two-year period, the pandemic has very strongly impacted the commuting landscape in the United States." Writing in a July 2023 report from *MIT Management, Sloan School* journal, we learn from Dylan Walsh that "The Bureau of Labor Statistics found that around 27% of U. S. workforce was working remotely at least part of the time as of August and September 2022, while a handful of academic surveys have suggested the number is closer to 50%."

The remarkable rise in suburban living has often necessitated the car as a means to get to work, shop, and entertain oneself and one's family, and although that model has spread to other parts of the world, Americans as a people still walk less than most of the rest of the world. Journalist Kea Wilson wrote in an April 2023 article "Exactly How Much Less America Walks Than Other Countries, In Five Charts" in *STREETSBLOGUSA*:

"Of the 11 countries in the sample for which data was available for all trip purposes, the U. S. tied last ... among the populations that walk for the lowest percentage of overall trips (12 percent)."

The author cites three additional hypotheses as to why Americans walk so little relative to other large, industrialized countries. They are:

- Lack of sidewalks and safe walking surfaces and conditions

- "Walkable places sell for a premium." That is, real estate is more expensive, as a rule, where walking conditions are feasible. The author says that "... for everyone else stuck in an autocentric place, walking is a mode of last resort."

- "Pedestrians die more on U. S. roads by every metric – and it's getting worse."

The confluence of all these factors – unabated American processed food consumption, the unstoppable rise in fast food, *a cultural acceptance of overweight/obesity*, a more sedentary populace – as well as the attitude among many that "a pill can handle my problems," has brought us to where we are today. And in addition to human suffering due to illness this is costing us and much of the rest of the world a ton of money.

But what of the economic impact in a huge country like the United States? According to a 2022 report from the CDC, obesity costs the US healthcare system about 173 billion USD a year. But October 2018 *Milken Institute* report by Hugh Waters and Marlon Graf ("America's Obesity Crisis, The Health And Economic Costs

Of Excess Weight") paints a more dire picture, revealing that in 2016, "chronic diseases driven by the risk factor of obesity and overweight accounted for 480.7 billion dollars in direct health care costs in the U.S., with an additional 1.24 trillion dollars in indirect costs due to lost economic productivity." Most impressively, they pointed out that "the total cost of chronic diseases due to American obesity and overweight was 1.72 trillion dollars – equivalent to 9.3 percent of the U. S. gross GDP" and that "obesity as a risk factor is by far the greatest contributor to the burden of chronic diseases in the U.S., accounting for 47.1 percent of the total cost of chronic diseases nationwide." I suspect the numbers are worse now relative to 2016, since the overweight/obesity rate has increased.

The picture globally is just as bleak. In Julia Belluz's "Report: Obesity could cost the world over $4 trillion a year by 2035" from *STAT News* (March 2023) the author quotes work from the World Obesity Federation, a partner of the World Health Organization. Her key findings were:

- over half the world will be overweight or obese by 2035

- if current trends continue, this may cost all of us 4.32 trillion dollars annually or 3 percent of global GDP

- no country has had a decline in obesity prevalence since 1975

- University of Sydney pediatrician and professor Louise Barr states "... more adolescents now enter adulthood with established risk factors for chronic disease – they're more likely to develop type 2 diabetes, or have heart disease risk factors or orthopedic problems, sleep apnea of fatty liver disease."

- the projections, gleaned from data in 161 countries, may be underestimated they may not consider the costs related to long-term disability care.

- the report neglects to consider the effect of "weight stigma, and its very real impact on the livelihood of people living with obesity, a penalty that's especially hard for women."

- the most significant cost increases are "projected for low- and middle-income countries, where obesity rates are growing fastest."

- the problem itself is not attracting enough global attention but might later when there is what one observer, Johanna Ralston (CEO of the World Obesity Federation), "an existential threat."

In the last section of this book, I will offer some ideas as to how we as a global community might tackle this issue.

## The National Security Impact And Our Military Preparedness

The effect of overweight/obesity from our bad food and lifestyle habits is affecting our military preparedness. *America Security Project*'s white paper from October 2023, entitled "Combating Military Obesity: Stigma's Persistent Impact on Operational Readiness," shows us the truth behind this sentiment. Citing a threat to our country's military "recruitment, readiness, and retention", the report, authored by Courtney Manning, found that:

- 68 percent of active-duty service members are overweight or obese.

- Obesity is the leading cause for military applicant disqualification, and "a primary contributor to in-service injuries and medical discharges."

- The rates of military obesity itself have more than doubled over ten years (10.4 percent in 2012 to 21.6 percent in 2022).

These are alarming statistics and are a direct result of the increase in overweight/obesity in our nation's young people. The unrestrained penetrance of UPF and sedentary lifestyles have been acutely expressed, it seems, among children and teens and now we are witness to a growing national security issue that seems to worsen with each passing year. From the *American Security Project's* "Briefing Note" by Matthew Wallin of March 2023, we see yet again the challenges our military is facing with regard to too high BMI. The author issued both a dire warning and wake-up call:

> "If trends in overweight and obesity continue, especially amongst the populations which are or will soon be within military service age, the military may not be able to recruit enough personnel to fulfill its national security obligations. Increasing reliance on a smaller number of combat-ready troops to secure U.S. policy objectives will place increased mental and physical wear on those forces, likely increasing overall attrition in the size of the force as those individuals exit the service."

The author of the article articulated various possible solutions to address this recruitment shortfall, including pre-induction mili-

tary fitness programs (like the Future Soldier Preparatory Course),
expanding of youth physical fitness programs in schools and by
local governments, treating obesity as a disease and boosting access
to relevant medical therapies, enhancing pharmacological treatment benefits coverage among medical plan insurers, and these
most important, grass-roots recommendations:

> "Expand the culture around fitness and nutrition,
> including through social media, technology and
> apps ... New thinking is needed about what motivates
> fitness and nutrition, and how technology, social media,
> and software can be used to encourage a culture of
> fitness ... Social media influencers may be a powerful
> help in improving public behavior around nutrition and
> exercise practices ... often by youth who are or will be in
> the target demographic for military recruiting."

# PART 4

## What do we do?

"If you wait until you're ready, you'll wait forever."
**Will Rogers, American entertainer**

So far I have attempted to give you an elementary but broad view of what bad food does to you and how the spread of UPF around the world has affected global health and well-being. Being but part of the story, bad diets combined with bad habits – like physical inactivity, substance abuse, and unregulated mental stress – augment each other in synergistic assaults on human physiology.

Ever since a flurry of scholarly articles, mainstream media coverage, and books on the danger of processed food (by authors such as David Kessler and Michael Moss) appeared a little a decade ago more attention has been paid to the matter but to apparently little avail. Rates of overweight/obesity continue their unhindered rise and the UPF makers reap ever-growing profits. Despite the drumbeat of warnings emanating from medical centers, medical schools, universities, government agencies and world health bodies, and think tanks all over the globe about the rising rates of obesity, cancer and cardiovascular disease in younger people, the costs in both human suffering and monetary capital and the generally bleak prospects for a quick solution remain. We in the medical community shake our heads as to the best course of action. After all, voices much more famous and influential than mine – think former FDA Commissioner David A. Kessler, University College London professor Chris Van Tulleken, and award-winning journalist Michael Moss – have all written excellent and in-depth books about the topic without inducing the necessary change to positively effect worldwide health.

Many people who follow this topic offer reasons why this is the case and I will now add my opinions to the chorus of those expressing their frustration and throwing their hands up in despair. Many of these ideas are not original by any means but they merit repeating – and tweaking. Many of you reading this may find that in my deviation from hard science in this section this discussion is based merely on opinion. But do realize I base these opinions – as a physician with 40 years in medicine – on a careful study of the literature, an understanding of the anatomy, physiology, and pathophysiology (biology of disease states) of the impact of higher body mass indexes, and as a careful student of patient – and therefore human – behavior.

The first and foremost of the challenges we face is a sociological one; the one I consider the most daunting to overcome. That is the issue of cultural enmeshment. By that I do not mean the more traditional use of the term, which can refer to "culture" as having to do with related ethnic or even racial groups. I mean something more subtle and insidious, more akin to sociological ingraining and an inability to look beyond oneself and see what the real truth is behind a given constellation of cultural norms. One of my favorite phrases in the world of philosophy comes from Arthur Schopenhauer, who famously said "Talent hits a target no one else can hit; genius hits a target no one else can see." And when it comes to "groupthink", whereby a group of individuals of any size accepts given norms and realities without the use of critical thought or the ability to consider alternatives, this becomes particularly perilous when addiction is added to the mixture. Since I contend that much of the weight and resultant health problems the world faces today is based on addiction, the additional parameters of groupthink mentality and cultural inability to "hit a target no one else can see", that is, to see the real impact of what your *individual* behavior is doing to your health due to prevailing attitudes and sentiment, is seemingly impossible to achieve.

I will give you an example. I grew up in, and live now in, one of *the* most affluent and well-educated counties in the United States – Montgomery County, Maryland. (My hometown of Bethesda is not only known as the home of the world-famous National Institutes of Health, Howard Hughes Medical Center, and Naval Support Activity Bethesda: Walter Reed, but also distinctive for the following demographics, as of 2017: according to the Bethesda Urban Partnership Bethesda's median household income is $154,559, of those 25 years of age and older the education attainment level of at least a Bachelor's degree is 83.7 percent, and the owner occupied housing unit rate is 67.3 percent.)

More broadly, according to DATAUSA the 2021 median household income in Montgomery County itself was $117,345, and the median property value was $508,600. The 2022 United States Census reported that 60 percent of Montgomery County residents 25 years of age and older have at least a bachelor's degree.

Despite this impressive array of statistics, when I talk to people in my community about the dangers of UPF to their health, they look at me as if I was speaking in tongues. I know that is a mere anecdotal allusion but these are not:

- According to a 2016 Montgomery County Maryland Government report entitled "Healthy Montgomery Core Measures", 58.7 percent of county residents were either overweight or obese.

- From 2018-2019, 22.4 percent of high school students were obese in Montgomery County and 56.4 percent of adults were either overweight or obese in Montgomery County in 2019, according to the report "2022 Montgomery County Hospital Collaborative Community Health Needs Assessment" on adventisthealthcare.com.

Although these metrics are lower than the national average, the idea that in a county as affluent, educated, and well-informed as Montgomery County, Maryland almost 6 out of 10 adult residents are either overweight or obese boggles my mind. To me this underlies a clear truth, and that is despite relative affluence and higher education, adults in Montgomery County, Maryland, and apparently elsewhere all over the world, are consistently and continually engaging in dietary and other behaviors that – because of higher BMIs – jeopardize their health. There are, I feel, multiple factors at play.

The reasons for failure in making a dent in the issue are many and, in my view, fall into these categories: the tight grip of addiction, the immense power of the UPF makers and big pharma, the "normalization" of obesity, the cost of healthy food and the presence of "food deserts", the issue of convenience and food preparation time constraints with regard to working people, health illiteracy, and patient mentality regarding medication versus lifestyle change. Before I offer possible solutions to overweight/obesity as a world health threat, I will cover the above-mentioned challenges first.

## Addiction

My position throughout this discourse has been that bad food causes an addiction, one that is apparently very hard to break. With the damage done to the hypothalamus some of the damage may be irreversible. However, due to persistent hypothalamic injury I am not surprised that overweight/obesity continues to rise in both the United States and around the world. A recent March 15, 2023, *WebMD* article by writer Brenda Goodman MA and reviewed by Poonam Sachdev, MD on the subject of food addiction expresses this sentiment perfectly. In that article the author discusses the addictive nature of foods heavy in sugar, fat and salt, and notes that, based on brain imaging studies, the addiction for this bad food is as strong in certain brain centers as those for cocaine and heroin. The author explains it beautifully:

> "Like addictive drugs, highly palatable foods trigger feel-good brain chemicals including dopamine. One you experience pleasure associated with increased dopamine transmission in your brain's reward pathway from

eating certain foods, you may quickly feel the need to eat again ... When you have food addiction, you lose control over your eating behavior and spend excessive amounts of time involved with food and overeating or anticipating the emotional effects of compulsive overeating."

This addictive effect has been proven in the laboratory using brain imaging and lends further support to the anatomical nature of the addiction. The abundance of diets, supplements, meal plans, exercise regimens, pharmaceuticals, surgical interventions, institutional programs, apps, and counseling professionals all attest to the extreme difficulty entailed in beating bad food addiction. And even for those who have successfully lost weight, ceasing the interventions that initially helped them take off the pounds, often result in a regaining weight lost.

## The power of UPF makers and big pharma

The combined financial might and lobbying powers of the UPF makers and the pharmaceutical industries rival those of the oil industry, tobacco makers, and alcoholic beverage industry. Earlier in the book I presented the financial projections in revenue relevant to the food industry and drug manufacturers and noted that these numbers run in the trillions of dollars. With war chests growing that large in the coming years one might expect to see an increase, not a diminution, in the lobbying power and advertising budgets for these industrial giants. *Statista* tells us that for the month of January 2023 alone, the food industry spent $440 million dollars for advertising, and that for the year 2022 "measured media spending in the United States food, beverage, and candy sector amounted to 7.5 billion U.S. dollars – with restaurants accounting for another nine billion." *Open Secrets* revealed that in 2022 the annual lobbying expenditures related to food processing and sales were approximately 27.5 million dollars.

In the pharmaceutical industry the numbers were even more impressive. Again it was *Statista* that reported that in 2021 the drug makers put out 6.88 billion dollars on direct-to-consumer advertising, a small rise relative to spending the prior year. They also indicated that in 2022, lobbying expenditures were 373.74 million dollars.

Both industries also give considerable amounts of money supporting political campaigns. With the combined moneys spent on advertising, lobbying and political campaigns here in the United States, it is not difficult to understand why we are all so inundated with messages from these behemoths to buy and use their products.

### The "normalization" of obesity

I speak of the widespread acceptance of a higher body mass index not as a judgment but as a material fact. As I have emphasized earlier in this book, *no one should be judged, insulted, denigrated, criticized, or discriminated against because of their body mass index.* That does not mean, however, that medical professionals like me can turn a blind eye as to what science shows regarding a high BMI, and what the ramifications for all of us and our planet are because of it. I have stated that while a certain level of personal responsibility is necessary to maintain health – just as brushing your teeth and flossing and taking a daily shower are good for your dental health and physical hygiene – taking ownership of your weight is not that simple. So important to global health is the issue of weight that the academic medical community, with regard to personal perceptions and high BMI, is taking careful and growing notice.

Writing in *Obesity* (the official journal of The Obesity Society) in July, 2018, Raya Muttarak in her article "Normalization of Plus Size and the Danger of Unseen Overweight and Obesity in England", the author expressed some fascinating findings prevalent in the study population:

"The persistence of the failure of individuals with overweight in recognition represents unsuccessful interventions of health professionals in tackling overweight and obesity. A close examination of demographic and socioeconomic characteristics associated with underestimation of weight status reveals social inequalities in weight misperception patterns . . . Likewise, the higher prevalence of overweight and obesity among individuals with lower levels of education and income may contribute to visual normalization, that is, more habitual visual exposure to people with excess weight than their counterparts with higher socioeconomic status . . ."

The author concludes by saying "The upward trend in underassessment of overweight and obesity status in England is possibly the result of the normalization of *overweight and obesity*" (italics mine).

This study is a valuable example of how persistent perceptions of cultural norms influence closed groups – in this case poorer members of native English and immigrant societies in England – and perpetuate the problem of overweight/obesity in given populations. In fact these same cultural norms appear to be expressed close to my home in Montgomery County, Maryland, where despite a more affluent and educated populace, weight problems persist, albeit to a lesser degree. To me, that reveals the strength of the addiction itself.

Continuing the theme of the normalization of high BMI, we find this issue insinuating itself into discussions in the mainstream media. There appears to be a small but growing backlash to the idea that an extremely high BMI is merely an acceptable personal choice and that the body positivity movement is just one of the many desirable social postures that should be embraced by society.

Writing in az*central* on April 13, 2016, journalist Linda Valdez's article "Valdez: C'mon people, stop normalizing obesity" said this:

> "Let's not normalize obesity. We should not be telling people it's OK to be fat based on some desire to make everybody love their body ... Spare me the homilies about 'body shaming'. No one's humanity should be judged on the basis of appearance ... We have done those things. And it was wrong ... We need to accept people as people. Not as body types. Fine ... But this is getting ridiculous ... The goal should be health ... Much of today's obesity epidemic in adults and children is caused by junk food and inactivity. These are not healthy habits. These habits – and the obesity they cause –should be called out and decried. We all have different body shapes, and I'm all for celebrating that. But pushing obesity a as new normal is not healthy for our minds or bodies."

Although I would have expressed it differently, the point comes across well enough. The only thing I would add to the article is that much of obesity, coming from a framework of addiction, is not the fault of the high BMI sufferer, but was imposed on that person when the eating of bad food began. We all know how difficult addictions are to break and placing full blame on the addicted is not constructive to finding the solution. But Valdez is right; the "high-BMI creep" we see in television ads, where many if not most of the actors portrayed, assuming the advertiser wanted to accurately represent a cross-section of America, are overweight or obese, is an apt indicator of the "normalization" she speaks of.

## The rising cost and relative scarcity of good food

Food that is good for you costs more, sometimes a lot more, than bad food. Perhaps in no time in modern history have calories coming from UPF and other bad food been so cheap. The 2013 news release "Eating healthy vs. unhealthy diet costs about $ 1.50 more per day" from Harvard's T. H. Chan School of Public Health, makes a compelling point:

> "Meta-analysis pinpoints the price difference of consuming a healthy diet, which could be a burden for low-income families but is trivial compared with health costs of eating an unhealthy diet."

The news release quotes researchers who suggest "that unhealthy diets may cost less because food policies have focused on the production of 'inexpensive, high volume' commodities, which has led to 'a complex network of farming, storage, transportation, processing, manufacturing, and marketing capabilities that favor sales of highly processed food products for maximal industry profit."

And we can see the truth in this every day in America, where you can get two double cheeseburgers, fries, and a 24-ounce soft drink for under 5 bucks at a fast-food joint – enough calories, saturated fat, and refined carbohydrate to last you multiple days – all in one meal.

The inability of many Americans, especially lower income groups, in securing healthy food at a price they can afford, is growing worse by the day. A lot of that has to do with the "maximal industry profit" mentioned in the article above, but there are other factors at play. From the *National Public Radio* Show "Morning Edition" on December 11, 2017, the segment "How Dollar General is Transforming Rural America", writer Frank Morris revealed the socioeconomic effects behind that store's wide presence in our nation's rural areas. He explains that when Dollar General moves into a rural community, local retailers and grocers may suffer because they cannot compete with the lower prices that Dollar General can offer with regard to many non-grocery and some less healthy, processed groceries. The NPR segment pointed out that:

> "Retail analyst Mike Paglia says the chain succeeds by selling everyday items at recession-era prices. 'In a lot of rural areas times are very, very, difficult, and a lot of shoppers are still struggling to get by,' Paglia says. Even before the recession, it was tough to run a store in rural America, according to Kent Baker, publisher of the *Moville Record* in Moville, Iowa. 'Half the grocery stores in Iowa closed between the years of 1995 to 2005,' he says."

The article emphasizes that when Moville "lost its last grocery store, locals fought back . . . the community donated roughly $600,000 in cash and property to build a new one. Then the residents enticed grocery owner Chet Davis . . . to take over the new store . . . 'We were doing real well, we were making a profit, and keeping our customers satisfied,' Davis says. 'Then in come Dollar General.' . . . In 2016, Dollar General built a location a stone's throw from Davis' store. Davis said his sales plunged about 30%, initially, and that Dollar General sells some items at a lower price than he can get them at wholesale."

The article goes on to say that the local grocers, at least at the time of the article, sold fresh meat and produce, items they claim were not available at Dollar General at the time. Store owners surveyed in the area, according to the article, have called "competition from Dollar General a top threat to small-town grocers."

Media reports have stated that Dollar General is now offering more produce to its consumers. The company announced recently that it will expand its offering of fresh produce from 3,000 to an additional 2000 of its 18,800 stores, according to journalist Michael Totty, writing in the *UCLA Anderson Review* March 8, 2023 article "Expanding chains drive out independent grocers, reduce access to fresh produce."

But besides "maximal industry profit" and the competitive advantage of the national chains over mom-and-pop grocery stores, there's politics. Well, politics and money, of course. And that is exactly what reporter Gene Baur was referring to in his July 2023 article in *Fortune* magazine entitled "Why is healthy food so expensive in America? Blame the Farm Bill that Congress always renews to make burgers cheaper than salads."

The crux of the article revolves around the power of agribusiness lobbyists here in Washington, DC, and their influence in getting the Farm Bill – a $700 billion expenditure over the next 5 years by the government – to "enrich themselves at the expense of agricultural communities, human health, animal welfare, and environmental sustainability."

The original idea of the bill was to help cash-strapped farmers during The Great Depression and Dustbowl eras. But Baur's analysis of the bill's consequence today is quite different than simply giving American farmers the help they need. Instead the result is that "Farm Bill policies have been hijacked, resulting in the demise of family farms, the proliferation of food that makes us sick, and widespread ecological destruction." He cites the heavy subsidies allotted to corn and soy, which are used to farm animals that will be used for meat on an industrial scale. Through this action the bill enables "the overproduction of fat-laden animal product s and highly processed foods, making unhealthy food cheap and accessible. This contributes to, according to Bauer, "heart disease and other chronic diet-related illnesses that cost our nation billions of dollars annually in preventable health care costs." He says that the funds in the Farm Bill programs should, in part at least, "be revised to incentivize fruits, vegetables, and other healthy foods and to make them more accessible and affordable." He mentions that 90 % of U. S. adults do not eat the nutritionists' recommended allowance of fruits and vegetables, and the scarcity in access to produce, especially in poorer communities.

## Time constraints and the convenience factor of bad food

In our fast-paced world it seems that everyone is in a hurry. And with good reason. Families have to rely more on two earners than one to make it in a highly inflationary economic environment. And the FIRE phenomenon (Financial Independence, Retire Early) whereby young earners want to save a large portion of their income in order to retire in their 30s or 40s has been popular among millennials. All of this is conducive to having access to meals that are quick, easy to prepare, and portable. The problem is that these types of meals are often not healthy simply because they may contain a fair amount of processed ingredients or might simply qualify as bad-for-you fast food itself.

From *Henry Ford Health* on September 23, 2023, came the article "Ultra-Processed Foods Are Sabotaging Your Diet: Here's How To Cut Them Out". In that article the author not only calls out the usual fast food and UPF food suspects that contribute to unhealthy eating, but vegan and vegetarian foods as well. This fact stood out:

> "Foods that are marketed to vegans, vegetarians and people following a gluten-free diet – including almond milk, alternative meat products and bakery items – are often full of gums, fillers, preservatives and other ingredients."

The partial fix, according to the article, is to

- Eat whole foods, like apples instead of applesauce and fresh nuts instead of a nutty granola bar.
- Eat more fruits and vegetables because we all need between five to nine servings a day. A handful of carrot sticks, cut celery or a pear is better than processed apple chips or processed potato chips.

- Examine the ingredient list. The shorter the better, and the more names of ingredients you can pronounce and recognize the better too.

- Shop for and carry foods with only one ingredient. It is easier, quicker, and healthier to bring an apple, a portion of fresh greens with olive oil and vinegar as dressing, some mixed nuts, pure dark chocolate, and a bottle of unsweetened iced tea to work than to travel to the fast-food place and load up on UPF and other saturated fat, refined carbohydrates, and sugar that's bad for you.

It takes creativity, thought, a little extra time, and a lot of "getting used to" to make these changes but in the long run they are worth it and will probably improve and extend your life.

## The effect of health illiteracy

Health illiteracy, in which people have very little understanding of medicine, basic anatomy and physiology, and healthcare policy, is rampant in America. In my 2021 book *What Your Doctor Won't Tell You* I quoted reporter Tina Trenker, who in 2011 (from an article on www.governing.com) gave a more technical definition of health illiteracy as, according to the US Department of Health and Human Services

" . . . the degree to which individuals have the capacity to obtain, process, and understand basic health information and services needed to make appropriate decisions. The percentage of the US population who can do so is shockingly low. Only 10 percent are fully literate when it comes to health instructions . . . Nearly 15 percent are totally health illiterate, mostly due to language barriers. . . The human cost is telling. . . Low health literacy is linked to higher rates of disease and mortality, as many as 100,00 deaths per year."

More recently, the US Department of Health and Human Services in their Healthy People 2030 initiative, confirmed that 90 percent of Americans have issues with health literacy, and that people with low health literacy "are more likely to have poorer health outcomes, including hospital stays and emergency room visits . . . make medication errors, have trouble managing chronic diseases, skip preventative services, like flu shots."

The precise degree to which health illiteracy contributes to the overweight/obesity epidemic is not known but I suspect that it is a major contributor. What I know for sure is that people all over the world – for the many reasons I have already discussed in this book – are neglecting the growing body of evidence that the consumption of UPF and other bad food is leading them to a life of chronic illness and premature death. Poor or rich, educated or not, there seems to be no discrimination here. The only difference is to what degree this effect occurs, not *that* it occurs. It is impossible to tease out how many individuals know that high BMI is a threat to their health and simply don't care versus those who know and do care but cannot, for some reason, effect the change necessary to improve the situation. Similarly we don't know how many people are oblivious to the deleterious effect on health that high BMI carries with it, and why is it that they apparently can't appreciate what should be fairly obvious to anyone who owns a body – the fatigue, being short winded when climbing a flight of stairs, the joint pain, the gastric reflux, the skin irritation and breakdown when body surfaces rub together, the inability to play with one's children without exhaustion – what the costs of high BMI entail. I appreciate the challenges and sympathize with the struggle and pain of those who deal with these issues and who cannot cause the change they would like to see, despite all their efforts. That is where the newer weight loss injectables may be lifesavers. But for the rest of the people who struggle with higher BMI and ignore the perils, I respectfully ask to take the evidence I've presented seriously and seek professional help.

## What have others suggested, and can it work?

We've examined the many roadblocks to progress and I am certain there are so many more that I have overlooked. But to find a way out of this quagmire is going to be extremely difficult and will take a lot of time, if it is possible at all. Whether one takes top-down approaches, such as legislative regulation, other government interventions, lawsuits, and concerted efforts from the medical community, or bottom-up efforts, like a push for greater personal responsibility, a social pushback against accepting overweight/obesity as the new normal, and grass-roots efforts to educate and inform the public about the dangers of UPF to health and resultant impact on the environment, we all have a very long way to go.

But there is hope, as evidenced by what happened in the tobacco industry, particularly with reference to cigarette smoking and what is happening now relevant to climate change. In part due to lawsuits and legislation against the Big Tobacco, cigarette smoking has fallen in America from about 43 percent of American adults in 1965 to just under 14 percent in 2018. A similar percentage drop in cigarette smoking has occurred in young people from 1991 to 2017. In January of 1971, cigarette advertisements were banned from television. Why not fast food today? With regard to climate change there are efforts now underway to hold oil companies accountable in courts of law for the environmental impact allegedly caused by their actions and products. *CNN* reporter Ella Nilsen wrote her January 8, 2024 article "Supreme Court decides to weigh in on Minnesota's climate lawsuit against big oil companies":

> "Besides Minnesota, California, other states and municipalities have sued big oil companies , in some cases asking courts to compel them to pay for abatement funds to help pay for damages from climate-fueled disasters like floods, wildfires, and extreme heat."

It is conceivable that groups or individuals will now bring lawsuits against the makers of UPF alleging that their products addicted them to dangerous products – similar to those in the Big Tobacco cases.

Governments have also weighed in on the issue. Van Tulleken points out that in Chile, which has some of the highest obesity rates in the world, officials in that country have become so alarmed that:

> "Chile implemented a set of policies that put marketing restrictions and mandatory black octagonal labels on foods and drinks high in energy, sugar, sodium, and saturated fat. These foods were also banned in schools and heavily taxed."

Can similar action be that far behind here in the United States? No one knows, but with lobbying power of the UPF makers, I would not hold my breath.

In his book *Ultra-Processed PEOPLE,* which I have quoted frequently in this work, Van Tulleken has offered some suggestions about how a dent can be made UPF's effect on our collective health. He has suggested, in my reading, that since the UPF makers are in the business of making money and answering to shareholders, self-regulation and self-governance in the industry is unlikely to result in much change. Indeed, he speaks of the fact that when it comes to people who purport to be concerned about the issue, "the lines between food activism and the UPF industry are also very blurred", at least when it comes to the state of affairs in the United Kingdom. I suspect it is not so different in other parts of the world. He does, however, offer these suggestions:

> "First, the people who make policy and inform policy should not take money directly or indirectly from the food industry. Second, the best way to increase rights and freedoms is to restrict marketing . . . Policymakers, and that includes doctors and scientists, need to see themselves as regulators . . . those who seek to limit the harms of these companies must have an adversarial relationship with them."

I could not agree more. The foxes should not, under any circumstances, be guarding the henhouse. (I would extend that thinking to drug company sponsorship of medical studies that involve their products.) Later in his discussion he emphasizes what I consider to be a basic truth: you cannot at the same time advocate for a solution to the problem while making money from the problem itself.

Former FDA director David Kessler has offered his own advice. In his *Young Reader's Edition* of his bestselling book *The End of Overeating* Kessler explains pragmatic ways that young people might break the bad food addiction. These include:

- Adopting new habits that will enable you to retrain your brain and enjoy "good food". By eating foods that are not UPF and foods laden with saturated fat, sugar, and refined carbohydrates you will eventually retrain yourself to like better-for-you foods.

- Bear in mind "to end overeating, remember the ways that sugar, fat, and salt make us feel bad." He wants us to focus on the fact that the food industry is trying to hook you, that these foods do not truly satisfy you, and that you need to look at food in a new way.

- Recognize the "food cues", the things that give you the urge to overeat. He advocates having "a plan for dealing with your cues" and getting support from family, friends, and professionals.

- Set rules for yourself regarding eating good food and getting adequate exercise.

- Learn to eat when you are hungry, enjoy your food while you eat it, and know when to stop. He says, "good eaters all have a plan for what, where, and how they will eat."

- Be patient and don't get down on yourself. Eating to break the addiction takes time.

Geared to a younger audience, these suggestions are applicable to all age groups and constitute a framework for responsible and sensible eating. They may sound simplistic and even trite, but they work.

These are two very different approaches to the problem. Van Tulleken's views were chosen to be representative of the "top-down" approach, and Kessler's the "bottom-up". But to really get a lasting solution will require combined efforts – from policy makers, activists, individuals, and most of all, the medical profession itself. That, combined with *a cultural shift in the way we view the issue of overweight/obesity and the food we eat,* is the only way, in my opinion, that we can achieve results. Without that, we are wasting our time.

The cultural shift I mention has to permeate society and can be best achieved in a backdrop of societal efforts and political legislation that attack the problem from many angles. This is the way we as a society brought smoking levels down so dramatically. Perhaps we need to tax bad food the way we tax cigarettes. Will restricting when and where advertisements can be aired make a difference? Do we need warning labels on UPF like the ones adopted in Chile?

And the dangerous politically correct posturing about the irrelevance of high BMI has got to stop. We need to call out high BMI – with respect and sensitivity – for what it truly is, a danger to health. We surely need to redirect funds allocated in the Farm Bill so that growers of fresh fruits and vegetables receive the subsidies they need to force down the price of these food groups. Public assistance money, particularly the federal SNAP (Supplemental Nutrition Assistance Program) which assists low-income households, needs better policing. The programmed is flawed, as evidenced by this statement from the *Physicians Committee for Responsible Medicine*:

"More than half of SNAP benefits are taken by retailers for meats, sweetened beverages, prepared foods and desserts, cheese, salty snacks, candy, and sugar. Just 23.9 percent go for fruits, vegetables, grains, nuts, beans, seeds, and spices."

That has got to change.

And what of the medical profession? Are we physicians really doing enough to make a difference? Are we moving toward the cultural shift we so desperately need? I think the answer is a clear "no". Some of this is our fault and some is not. Let me tell you why.

First, we in healthcare have to lead by example. Pamela Peake M.D., M.P.H., writes in the *AMA Journal of Ethics* that 44 percent of doctors are overweight and 6 percent are obese and that *The Nurses Health Study* reports that 28 percent of nurses are overweight and 11 percent are obese. Studies mentioned in the article revealed that patients trusted the opinions of obese physicians less than if the physician was not obese.

Second, the practice model of much of Western medicine is completely backwards, focusing not on prevention but primarily on therapy for existing diseases. This *allopathic model* dominates medicine in the United States and many parts of the E.U. and the U.K. and relies on the concept that medication, surgery, and procedures are the mainstay therapeutic interventions needed to foster health and health maintenance. In my view this "band-aid on a cut" approach is all wrong – why not avoid the cut to begin with instead of covering it up? Why isn't patient counseling, education, and a strong emphasis on prevention the primary focus, instead of the mere stamping out of medical fires that so many of my colleagues complain about?

I'll tell you why. Time. That, and patient expectations.

Let's talk about time, or the lack of it. Because of the shortage of physicians and other healthcare workers, healthcare providers are overburdened and overwhelmed. The growing number of chronically sick patients is pushing the healthcare system in the direction of partial collapse. A *Medscape Physician Compensation Report* from 2017 revealed that the average time a primary care family physician spent with a patient was in the range of 13-16 minutes. Some physicians in that class reported a longer time frame of 17-24 minutes. But I think my point is made. That is not enough time to obtain a proper patient history, do a thorough physical exam, review the patient's medications, lab tests and other studies, discuss the risks and benefits of treatment options, and counsel the patient on effective preventative measures, all within the framework of the widespread health illiteracy I referenced earlier.

And patient expectations come into play as well. Patients foster the all too prevalent attitude that a pill will solve their problems faster, better, and with less effort, than anything they can personally do to improve the situation. Part of that is just human nature, and part is the fault of the drug companies and their advertising efforts. What immediately pops into my mind is the television ad showing a high BMI construction worker smiling in the knowledge that he can enjoy his chili dog without the fear of heartburn because of his antacid pill. Did he think maybe that if he didn't eat that garbage he wouldn't need the pill, and the side effects that go along with it, in the first place? This attitude, so common among all of us, is the reason why we continue to be sick and overmedicated. The band-aid instead of preventing the cut in the first place.

Finally, we have to foster efforts in schools that will not only rid them of vending machines that sell UPF and sodas but teach and reinforce beneficial basic nutrition and physical fitness habits starting at a very young age. This is so difficult to do but so worth it in the long run. We must influence people when they are young if we have a shot at making a difference. It worked with smoking, and it can work with bad food as well.

# CLOSING THOUGHTS

"It does not require many words to speak the truth."

**Chief Joseph, Nez Perce Tribe**

People ask me why I am so passionate about the issues we have discussed. The answers, which are easy for me to produce, are twofold. The first is that bearing witness to my late sister Lisa's suffering who, at the age of seven was stricken with a disease the development of which she had no hand in, gave me firsthand knowledge of what damage metabolic disease can do. Consider this:

On New Year's Eve, December 31, 1981, almost a year before her death, my sister Lisa lay in bed in my parents' home, blind, in pain, partially deaf, covered in scars, bearing a sallow complexion, and with a malfunctioning donated kidney. My parents had gone out for the evening. I had been invited to a New Year's Eve party in Bethesda and Lisa, I knew, would be all alone that night. I asked her if she wanted me to skip the party and stay with her and she said, her blind stare gazing into unseen space, "No mister" (she often called me mister), you go have a good time." My tears fell from my face onto her bedclothes. I was torn. I asked again but she insisted I go. That was about the worst few minutes I ever felt in my life. While most people her age were out having a good time, she sat alone, suffering from a disease that would never get better. Eleven months later she was gone.

Second, for almost 40 years as a doctor, I have seen patients suffer the dramatic effects of adult metabolic disease – sometimes due to ignorance and oftentimes due to their own behavior – that have struck me as so unnecessary. This is not a judgment; it is mere observation based on long and wide experience.

The world has changed in so many ways in the last fifty years, and much of it for the worse. The planet is more and more the victim of climate change, wars rage more ominously across the globe, and economic inequality has worsened. So too with human health. I challenge anyone over the age of 50 in our country to turn to his or her high school yearbook and look at the faces and physiques of your former classmates. Look at the movies, television shows, and advertisements from the years preceding the 1980s and witness how higher body mass indexes, so relatively uncommon back then, have become the new normal. This too is not judgment, but merely fact.

You have now read the science behind my arguments, as well as the social and economic constructs that are a significant part of the story. You have also read of the possible remedies proposed, many of them from distinguished physicians and medical experts with far more clout than I have. Am I optimistic about the future health of the nation, and indeed the world? Unfortunately, I am not.

Why? Because I am first and foremost a realist. The powers that are joined against solutions are just too strong, in my opinion. Money, the driver behind the story I have told, is a force too great to overcome. The makers of UPF, junk food, *bad food* – and

Big Pharma – are just too powerful to take on, unlike a singular industry like Big Tobacco. Everyone knew deep down that smoking was bad for you, even the makers of the cigarettes themselves. But food is another issue altogether. The makers of UPF tout the convenience, price, and abundance of their products as evidence of their wide appeal and benefit. They say that without their products a great number of people all over the world will not be able to feed themselves and many would have to go hungry. And that is difficult to refute, as painful as that is to admit.

And then there is that old enemy addiction. Yes, people were able to overcome their addiction to cigarettes through a number of means; "cold turkey", nicotine gum, anti-depressants, cognitive behavioral therapy, hypnosis, unaffordability, you name it. They all played a part. But UPF is a different animal. Everyone has to eat, but not everyone has to smoke.

And that brings us to perhaps the most frightening aspect of all – the future inability of health care systems to deal with what is coming.

Part of the health illiteracy I spoke of is not being aware of the shortages coming very soon, as well as the changing demographics. According to the World Health Organization, by 2030 1 out of every 6 persons will be 60 or older, up from 1 billion people in 2020 to 1.4 billion people in 2030. According to the *Georgetown University Center for Retirement Initiatives*, the number of Americans 65 years of age and older was 49.2 million in 2016 and will grow to 74 million by 2030. At the present rate that will mean a daunting number of potentially chronically ill people will need medical care.

And now comes the really bad news. Who is going to care for all these people? Where will the money come from? In their 2020 book *Better Health Care Through Math, Bending the Access and Cost*

*Curves*, authors Sanjeev Agrawal and Mohan Giridharadas lay it on the line:

- By 2030, the number of adults sixty-five years of age or older will exceed the number of children eighteen years or younger in the United States.

- Older people have more chronic disease. By 2025, nearly 50 percent of the population will suffer one or more chronic diseases that will require ongoing medical intervention. This will . . . create a ballooning demand for healthcare services.

- The healthcare system as a whole is under tremendous financial strain . . . Health insurance premiums have increased 54 percent in the past ten years . . . And as the number of older Americans outstrips the number of younger Americans, the burden of paying for the system will fall increasingly on the smaller number of young people.

- The Association of American Medical Colleges projects that by 2032, there will be 122,000 too few physicians. By that year the shortage of nurses will be well over half a million.

The present state of American health and American healthcare, like it is in much of the world, is untenable. We cannot continue down this path. The time to act as to how we eat, move our bodies, and approach our physical, mental, and emotional health is well past due. We all have a lot of work to do.

# GLOSSARY

**Body mass index, or BMI,** is defined as a person's weight divided by the square of their height.

**Cytokines** are protein molecules that play a central role in immunity, inflammation, and autoimmune disease and are significant for their ability to tell other cells within the bloodstream how to fight infectious agents and other intruders.

**Glycemic index, or GI,** is a measure of how rapidly certain foods can make your blood sugar rise. Glycemic load, or GL, represents how much the ingested food will increase a person's serum glucose level after eating.

**Glycogen** is the body's storage form of glucose.

**Hormones** are chemical messengers released by the endocrine glands, like the thyroid gland, pituitary, pancreas, and adrenal glands, that are involved in specific bodily functions.

**Insulin** is the essential hormone that regulates blood sugar and is crucial to many metabolic functions.

**Neurotransmitters** are chemical messengers released by nerves to other nerves or tissues in the body in order to affect a certain function or physiologic response. The four neurotransmitters most well-known are acetylcholine, dopamine, serotonin, and glutamate. Adrenaline (epinephrine), gamma aminobutyric acid (GABA) and oxytocin are also neurotransmitters, each with specific functions.

**Oxidative stress** refers to an abnormal relationship between production and accumulation of reactive oxygen species or forms of oxygen molecules that are produced as byproducts of metabolism.

Refined carbohydrates are simple carbohydrates like glucose, sucrose and others sugars as well as grains that have their fibrous elements removed.

**Saturated fats** are those whose fatty acid chains have single chemical bonds. High consumption of these have been correlated to cardiovascular diseases and other diseases.

# ACKNOWLEDGMENTS

I would like to express my thanks to my publisher Maryann Karinch for her support in this project. I am grateful to Laura Belt and Dr. Ronald Kotler for bringing valuable research and articles to my attention. Thanks also go out to Gina Cavallaro for the information she gave me on the issue of weight and military preparedness. Thank you, Kim Abraham, for your valued thoughts on the cover art. And to my late father, Max G. Sherer M.D., thank you for being such a great medical teacher. I hope there is good golf wherever you are.

# AUTHOR BIO

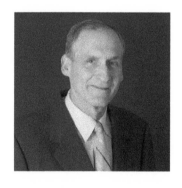 **DAVID SHERER, M.D.** is a recognized expert in health and medicine safety. He is a former member of Leading Physicians of the World, and a multi-time winner of Health-Tap's leading anesthesiologists award. Dr. Sherer has retired from his clinical anesthesiology practice in the suburbs of Washington, DC and now focuses on patient education, writing and patient advocacy; including as a medical and health video commentator for Bottom Line Inc.'s "What Your Doctor Isn't Telling You" columns and podcasts. Dr. Sherer is a tireless advocate for hospitalized patients, and believes that individual responsibility, and not government intervention, is the key to improving the general health and wellbeing of all Americans.

He is also the author of HOSPITAL SURVIVAL GUIDE, WHAT YOUR DOCTOR ISN'T TELLING YOU, and the novel INTO THE ETHER, also published by Armin Lear Press.

Milton Keynes UK
Ingram Content Group UK Ltd.
UKHW042317240324
439966UK00004B/437

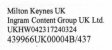

9 781963 271096